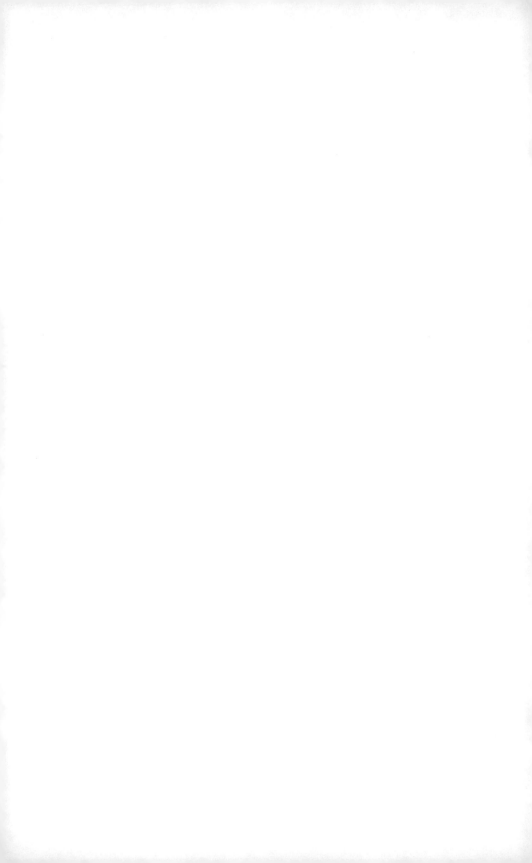

BUBONIC PLAGUE IN

NINETEENTH-CENTURY CHINA

Bubonic Plague in Nineteenth-Century China

CAROL BENEDICT

STANFORD UNIVERSITY PRESS

STANFORD, CALIFORNIA

Stanford University Press
Stanford, California
© 1996 by the Board of Trustees of the
Leland Stanford Junior University
Printed in the United States of America

CIP data are at the end of the book

Stanford University Press publications are
distributed exclusively by Stanford
University Press within the United States,
Canada, Mexico, and Central America;
they are distributed exclusively by
Cambridge University Press throughout
the rest of the world

To the memory of George M. Benedict

Acknowledgments

I WOULD LIKE to thank the many teachers, colleagues, friends, and family members who have generously contributed to the effort that produced this study. My doctoral dissertation advisors, Harold Kahn and Lyman Van Slyke, not only enthusiastically supported and encouraged me through the many phases of this project but also provide continued inspiration as rigorous scholars, gifted teachers, and caring persons. I am also indebted to Ann Janetta, Nathan Sivin, and Susan Naquin for their extensive and probing comments on the dissertation. Although I was unable to incorporate all their suggested revisions, the final product is undoubtedly richer because of their efforts.

I have received financial support from a number of institutions. Funding for research in China was provided by a grant from the Committee on Scholarly Communication with the People's Republic of China. Dissertation writing was made possible by a fellowship from the Mrs. Giles Whiting Foundation. Final revisions and manuscript preparation were undertaken during a research leave funded by the National Endowment for the Humanities, the Chiang Ching-Kuo Foundation, and Williams College. Georgetown University provided subventions for map preparation. I am grateful to all these institutions for the assistance they provided.

My year of research in China was rendered more enjoyable and productive by the help provided by the Ministry of Public Health, the Beijing College of Traditional Medicine, and particularly by my research advisor, Professor Zhen Zhiya. Special thanks are also due to

Dr. Tian Jingguo of the Yunnan Branch of the China Medical Association. I would also like to thank the reference and circulation staffs of the Library of the National Academy of Traditional Chinese Medicine, the First Historical Archives, the Peking Union Medical School Library, the National Minorities Institute Library, the Beijing National Library, and the Beijing Capitol Library. Nor could this research have been completed without the assistance of the librarians and staff of the East Asian Collection of the Lou Henry Hoover Library at Stanford University, the East Asian Division of the Library of Congress, and the interlibrary loan staff of Sawyer Library at Williams College.

Many other friends and colleagues have made invaluable contributions to this project. Bryna Goodman, Evelyn Rawski, and Marta Hanson carefully went through early versions of the manuscript and made thorough, insightful, and helpful suggestions for its improvement. James Lee and Chang Chia-feng generously shared their unpublished work with me. Others who assisted in various ways are George T. Crane, Neil Diamant, Peter Frost, Charlotte Furth, Paul Howard, Iijima Wataru, Paul Katz, Tom Kohut, Norman Kutchner, Angela Leung, Melissa Macauley, Joyce Madancy, Susan Mann, James Millward, John Shepard, G. William Skinner, and Kevin Scott Wong. Special thanks are due to Ch'en Ch'iu-kun, Yue Mingbao, and Adam Chau for draft translations of selected materials. Amy Klatzkin skillfully guided me through the editorial and production process; Victoria Scott carefully and meticulously copyedited the final manuscript.

I am profoundly grateful to my family and friends, and particularly to my parents, Muriel and James Benedict. To my friends in Beijing, Lin Qiang, Lu Yumin, and Wan Jun, I owe more than I can say. Palle Henckel offered endless good humor and indispensable computer advice. Michelle Vaughen and Niels Crone saw me through the final phases of this project and the gestational stages of a new one. Appreciation is extended to my colleagues in the History Department and the Asian Studies Program at Williams College for their immense collegiality and for the high standards they set as teacher-scholars. Cathy Johnson, Alison Case, and Scarlett Jang provided both criticism and companionship in our Friday afternoon sessions. Finally, Paul Ashin—through the years and across the miles—has always been there to advise, to critique, and to read yet another draft. I owe my greatest debt to him.

Contents

Illustrations

MAPS

Tables

A Note on Translations,
Transliteration, Names, and Places

ALL TRANSLATIONS are by the author unless otherwise indicated. *Pinyin* is used for the transliteration of Chinese terms. The names of writers who publish in Chinese or Japanese appear in Chinese or Japanese form, with surname preceding given name. I have retained each author's preferred form of transliteration and name order for authors who publish in English, presenting Chinese and Japanese names in Western fashion only if the author does so as well. (Virtually all such authors thus appear with surname first in in-text references. A comma appears in the Works Cited because I treated these authors like all others writing in English.)

The Chinese words for jurisdictional names have been translated as follows: *fu* is rendered as "prefecture," *ting* as "subprefecture," *zhou* as "department," *xian* as "county," and *si* as "township." The terms *zhili ting* and *zhili zhou* have been translated as "autonomous subprefecture" and "autonomous department"; *tuzhou* and *tusi* are rendered as "minority department" and "minority township." The terms *xian* and *zhou* are appended to place names when the name would otherwise be monosyllabic. Chinese sources seldom distinguish between the jurisdictional capital and the hinterland when referring to the territorial extent of epidemics. Where such distinctions are possible, they are indicated by the appropriate jurisdictional specification (city, county, etc.).

I generally use nineteenth-century names for places: thus Liaoning provice is termed Fengtian, Hebei province is called Zhili, and so forth. While most place names are those current during the Qing period, there are a number of exceptions. To avoid confusion, the city of Shenyang, known during the Guangxu period (1875–1908) as Fengtian, has been rendered as Shenyang throughout. I have retained the English forms of Canton, Macao, and Hong Kong for the cities of Guangzhou, Aomen, and Xianggang, respectively. The English names of treaty ports are provided at the first mention in the text of the Chinese name and in Character List B. Any other exceptions are also noted in the text and in Character List B.

Weisheng is translated as "sanitary" rather than its modern equivalent of "sanitation" or "hygiene." Although this translation is sometimes awkward, it follows nineteenth- and early-twentieth-century conventions and refers to public health as well as to sanitation and hygiene. Early-twentieth-century Sanitary Departments (*Weisheng si*) oversaw all aspects of public health and sanitation, including, for example, smallpox inoculations and street cleaning. Retaining the term "sanitary" serves to emphasize the multiple functions of such agencies.

Abbreviations

THE FOLLOWING abbreviations are used in citations in the text and notes. Works not listed here are cited in the text and notes by author and date; complete information for such works can be found in Works Cited, pp. 213–29.

GZD I   *Gongzhongdang, Zhupi zouzhe, Wenjiao lei, yiyao weisheng* (Imperially rescripted palace memorials, Culture and education category, Medicine and health subcategory). First Historical Archives, Beijing.

GZD II   *Gongzhongdang, Zhupi zouzhe, Neizheng lei, zhenji* (Imperially rescripted palace memorials, Internal administration category, Relief subcategory). First Historical Archives, Beijing.

NA   National Archives of the United States, Washington, D.C. *National Archives files and microfilm publications are cited as follows:*

   PHS, RG 90   Public Health Service. Record Group 90. Central File, 1900.

   USDS, RG 59   Department of State. Record Group 59. General Records of the Department of State, Decimal File, 1910–29.

      M100   *Despatches of the United States Consuls in Amoy, 1844–1906.* Microfilm Publication 100.

      M101   *Despatches of the United States Consuls in Canton, 1790–1906.* Microfilm Publication 101.

      M105   *Despatches of the United States Consuls in Foochow, 1897–1901.* Microfilm Publication 105.

      M108   *Despatches of the United States Consuls in Hong Kong, 1844–1906.* Microfilm Publication 108.

NCH   *North China Herald.* 1894, 1911.

SYLXS   Chinese Academy of Medical Sciences, Institute for Research on Infectious and Parasitic Diseases. 1982. *Zhongguo shuyi liuxingshi* (The history of the spread of plague in China). 2 vols. Beijing.

BUBONIC PLAGUE IN
NINETEENTH-CENTURY CHINA

Introduction

OUTBREAKS OF bubonic plague have reached pandemic proportions on only three occasions in recorded history. The first was the plague of Justinian, which spread through the Middle East and the Mediterranean in the sixth century C.E. (Dols 1977: 14–19; Hirst 1953: 10). The fourteenth-century "Black Death" was the second. Beginning in 1347, plague spread from western Asia to the Middle East and the Mediterranean before moving on to Spain and France, finally reaching England, Scandinavia, Germany, and Poland (Benedictow 1992; Dols 1977; Shrewsbury 1970; Ziegler 1969). The third pandemic, which emerged at the end of the nineteenth century, vastly exceeded the first two in geographical scope. In 1894 bubonic plague appeared in Canton and Hong Kong. Within a few years the disease had spread from Hong Kong throughout much of Asia, reaching India in 1896, Vietnam in 1898, and Japan in 1899 (Hirst 1953: 104; Janetta 1987: 194; Velimirovic 1972: 493). By 1900 the international shipping trade had carried plague from Asia to global ports as far-flung as San Francisco and Glasgow, precipitating the pandemic that lasted well into the twentieth century (Hirst 1953: 296–303).

This modern pandemic had its origins in southwestern China. In the late eighteenth century an epidemic of bubonic plague broke out in Yunnan province. The earliest recorded epidemic of what may have been plague began in Yunnan in the 1770's. Between 1772 and 1830 the disease spread slowly from Yunnan's western frontier to the more populated areas in the center and southeast of the province. After

1830 plague subsided for a time, but then it reappeared in the mid-nineteenth century. This time it moved further east, spreading first through Guangxi and western Guangdong in the 1860's and 1870's and eventually reaching the Pearl River Delta in the 1890's. The disease also diffused farther up the Chinese coastline and across the Taiwan Straits, spreading to Fujian, Taiwan, parts of Zhejiang, and coastal cities such as Shanghai and Yingkou (Newchang).

The history of the third plague pandemic outside of China is well documented. Historians have written extensively about the plague in India, for example, examining its demographic effects (Klein 1986: 725–54; 1988: 723–55), the political conflicts it engendered within various branches of the British colonial government and the Indian National Congress (Catanach 1983: 216–43; 1987: 198–215; 1988: 149–71), and the popular Indian response to colonial medicine and public health (Arnold 1988: 391–426; Arnold 1993: 200–239; Chandavarkar 1992: 203–40). There are a number of histories of the modern plague in other countries, such as Indonesia (Hull 1987: 210–34). Still other works focus on the eclipse of grass-roots management of plague control in San Francisco by the United States Public Health Service and on the racially based public-health policies that emerged in the wake of plague outbreaks in South Africa and the United States (Kraut 1994: 78–96; McClain 1988: 447–513; Risse 1992: 260–86; Swanson 1977: 387–410; Trauner 1978: 70–87). In addition, the significance for biomedical plague research of the 1894 outbreak in Hong Kong and Canton has been investigated (Cunningham 1992: 209–44; Hirst 1953: 106–20).

Although a number of studies touch on the late-Qing plague epidemics in China, they do so only within the broader context of the worldwide pandemic (Hirst 1953: 101–4; Simpson 1905: 48–66; Wong and Wu 1935: 506–19; Wu 1936: 15–31).[1] Interested primarily in tracking the global diffusion of plague, these scholars made little effort to understand the history of the disease in China itself. Plague passed through a very large area of the country, but the complete extent of its territorial spread has remained undocumented. Nor has anyone analyzed how the Chinese tried to cope individually or communally with the crisis provoked by this disease.

This book looks at the Chinese origins of the modern plague pandemic in terms not of its effects elsewhere but of its causes and consequences within China. On the most general level, I seek to document as fully as possible the historical, geographical, epidemiological, and social dimensions of plague in late Qing China. More specifically, I address questions surrounding the origins of this disease in Yunnan; the reasons for its spread from the southwest to provinces lying along the southeastern seaboard; and the changing social, medical, and religious responses of the Chinese to it over the course of the nineteenth and early twentieth centuries.

The foregoing concerns shape the division of this work into six substantive chapters. Chapters 1, 2, and 3 employ a regional systems approach to establish a framework for understanding plague's intra-regional and interregional diffusion. Chapter 1 focuses on the plague's origins in southwestern China and offers an analysis of how economic growth in the eighteenth century produced ecological changes that precipitated the initial outbreaks in Yunnan. I show that plague was not a sign of economic collapse or demographic decline but a consequence of extensive development of China's southwestern frontier in the eighteenth century. Chapter 2 discusses the long-distance spread of the disease along nineteenth-century trade routes, particularly those used to transport domestically grown opium between Yunnan and the Lingnan region. Chapter 3 offers some tentative conclusions about plague's demographic effects, based on urban and rural patterns of plague diffusion in the Southeast Coast macroregion.

The final three chapters are concerned with the political and social dimensions of the late Qing epidemics. Chapter 4 is a survey of the etiological theories and religious interpretations that informed nineteenth-century medical, ritual, and administrative activity during epidemics generally. Chapter 5 provides a case study of plague in Canton and Hong Kong in 1894 and chronicles the conflicts that emerged between Chinese elite activists and the British colonial government over the proper way to respond to the epidemic. Chapter 6 describes changes in state and societal responses to epidemic plague in the final decade of Qing rule and details the central role plague played in the creation of Chinese state medicine and institutions of public health during the New Policies period (1901–11). I argue that, in contrast to Europe, the Qing state did not impose forceful public-health measures on society. This changed, however, as Western concepts of state medicine began to be accepted and adopted within China from the turn of the twentieth century on, largely as a consequence of the international politics of health surrounding the third pandemic.

The Epidemiology of Plague

The word "plague," as used here, refers to a specific disease described by modern biomedicine.[2] The causative organism, *Yersinia pestis* (sometimes called *Pasteurella pestis*), is a bacillus, some strains of which are quite harmful to humans. Its effects on humans, however, are incidental; plague is a zoonotic disease that primarily affects rodents and other animals. Animals and humans contract the infection from the bites of insects, usually rat fleas. The disease is only directly communicable if plague bacteria get into the lungs and the victim develops secondary pneumonia, thereby coughing up blood or respiratory droplets containing *Yersinia pestis*. This rare form of plague is highly contagious and invariably fatal within one or two days if not treated. In the more common bubonic form, bacteria attack the lymphatic system and highly visible "buboes" form in the groin, armpits, or neck two or three days after infection. Other symptoms include high fever, shivering, vomiting, headaches, giddiness, and delirium. Treatment with antibiotics in the early stages is now quite effective, but left untreated, bubonic plague kills 60 to 90 percent of those infected within five days. Other clinical forms of plague that occur less frequently include meningeal plague (affecting membranes of the brain and spinal cord) and septicaemic plague (affecting the circulatory system).

Plague currently persists among wild mammals living in certain well-defined geographical areas around the globe. Designated as "natural plague reservoirs" or "sylvatic plague foci," these wilderness areas have climatic and entomological features that support continued *Yersinia pestis* infection in animals. The number of animals that can serve as hosts for the infection in these natural reservoirs is quite large and by no means limited to rats. Marmots, ground squirrels, prairie dogs, rabbits, gerbils, mice, voles, and shrews can all harbor the disease. Natural plague foci are typically inhabited by several disparate species, each with its own level of resistance to plague. Those species that are highly resistant to plague infection maintain enzootic pools of *Yersinia pestis* bacteria because plague kills only a few animals each season. The rest of the population is immune to the disease and continues to carry infected fleas without adverse effect. When such fleas bite members of species that *are* susceptible, large numbers of the new hosts become infected and many die in episodes known as "epizootics." Fleas then abandon the carcasses in search of new hosts, including humans if they are nearby.

The transfer of plague from animals to humans occurs more frequently with some species than others. The most common agents in human plague transmission in European history were the black rat (*Rattus rattus*, sometimes called the ship rat) and the common brown rat (*Rattus norvegicus*, or the Norway rat). Brown rats and black rats now live virtually everywhere around the world. In addition, there are more than two hundred other rodent species that serve as vectors for human plague (Ji Shuli 1988: 480). Other animals, such as house cats, have also been implicated in the transfer of plague from rodents to humans. When ongoing plague infections are found among rats or domestic animals, a "commensal plague focus" is said to exist.

Humans come into contact with infected fleas when they encroach on an area where plague is enzootic or when infected animals move into or are brought into areas of human settlement. Fleas cannot jump far by themselves, but they can be passively transported by animal hosts that cover long distances (birds, rabbits, hares, and predators that feed on dead rodents) or by humans (in their baggage, in commercial goods, and in transport vehicles). The passive transport of infected fleas by people is the most common way plague is conveyed between human settlements. Fleas are carried along in a wide variety of commodities: raw cotton, wool, grain, and even in gunny sacks. Because people play an important role in the long-distance movement of infected fleas, plague tends to spread along transportation routes.

The Ecology of Plague in Present-Day China

Several of the world's natural plague reservoirs are located within the People's Republic of China. Pockets of enzootic foci now exist in 17 of China's 26 provinces (including Taiwan) and autonomous regions, affect 194 counties, and cover an area of about 500,000 square kilometers (Ji Shuli 1988: 64–66, 475). Chinese epidemiologists have typed ten different natural plague reservoirs, based on geographical location, the species of animal involved in maintaining the infection, and the particular strain of *Yersinia pestis* present (Table 1). There are more than fifty known plague-carrying mammals living in these ten areas, some forty different insect vectors, and seventeen unique strains of plague (ibid.: 479–80).

This book focuses on the three natural plague reservoirs in China that have posed a significant risk to human life in the past two hundred

6   Introduction

TABLE 1
Natural Plague Reservoirs in China

Location	Primary host(s)
The Qinghai and Tibetan Plateau	*Marmota himalayana* (Himalayan marmot)
Tianshan Mountains (Xinjiang)	*Marmota baibacina* (Bobak marmot)
	Citellus undulatus (long-haired souslik)
Pamir Plateau (Xinjiang)	*Citellus undulatus* (long-haired souslik)
Hulun Nur Plateau (Mongolia)	*Marmota sibirica* (Siberian marmot)
	Citellus dauricus (Daurian ground squirrel)
Manchurian Plain	*Marmota sibirica* (Siberian marmot)
	Citellus dauricus (Daurian ground squirrel)
Gan-Ning Loess Plateau	
(Gansu and Ningxia)	*Citellus alaschanicus* (Alashan souslik)
Inner Mongolian Plateau	*Meriones unguiculatus* (Mongolian gerbil)
Shiliyn Bogd Uul Plateau	
(Inner Mongolia)	*Microtus brandtii* (Brandt's vole)
Western Yunnan Transverse Valley	*Eothenomys miletus* (Oriental vole)
	Apodemus chevrieri (field mouse)
Southern China Commensal Rat	
Plague Focus (western Yunnan,	
Leizhou Peninsula, southern	
Fujian)	*Rattus flavipectus* (yellow-chested rat)

SOURCE: Ji Shuli 1988: 65–66.

years: the Manchurian Plain, the Western Yunnan Transverse Valley, and the Southern China Commensal Rat Plague Focus.[3] Most of the other reservoirs listed in Table 1 are in isolated regions of the country and thus pose little threat to humans. In these remote areas plague is only transferred to people when they actively invade the animals' wild habitat, for example, by hunting or trapping. Such cases are extremely rare. In contrast, on the densely populated Manchurian Plain, the disease can be easily transferred from the Daurian ground squirrel (*Citellus dauricus*) to the brown rat (*Rattus norvegicus*), the most common commensal rodent in northern China. This particular ecology of enzootic plague in northeastern China is the reason human plague has occurred frequently in Manchuria since at least the early twentieth century (Wu 1926; 1936).

The Western Yunnan Transverse Valley plague reservoir covers some 230 square miles in the Hengduan Mountains of southwestern China. Two plague-resistant species of wild animals in this mountainous region, the Oriental vole (*Eothenomys miletus*) and a kind of field mouse (*Apodemus chevrieri*), maintain ongoing enzootic infections. The area is also inhabited by the yellow-chested rat (*Rattus flavipectus*), a semiwild rodent that is highly susceptible to the particular strain of plague present among the *Eothenomys miletus* and the *Apodemus chevrieri* species. Plague is continually transmitted from the wild animals to this rat, which then carries the disease back to human settlements located near the wilderness area.

The yellow-chested rat (*Rattus flavipectus*) is by far the most common rodent found in southern China, and it is the reason plague persists even today (1) in areas of western Yunnan (the Western Yunnan Transverse Valley), and (2) on the Leizhou Peninsula and in southern Fujian (collectively termed the Southern China Commensal Rat Plague Focus).[4] It is classified by zoologists as a semiwild rat because it prefers to live in the upper stories or roofs of houses, but it can also live in vegetable gardens, fields, or the bush. It eats almost anything but prefers grain, beans, and other vegetable matter. During the harvest season it lives outside and eats ripe grain; most of the rest of the year it is found in human shelters. Although its natural habitat lies in provinces below the Yangzi River (and it is especially common in Yunnan, Guangxi, Guangdong, Fujian, Zhejiang, and Anhui), it has also been found in trucks and ships transporting goods to the north. The *Xenopsylla cheopis* (the Asiatic rat flea) is the most common rat flea in southern China and is the primary vector of plague transmission between the yellow-chested rat and humans.

The Historiography of Plague in Pre-Qing China

Even though, in modern biomedicine, the term "plague" refers specifically to the infection caused by *Yersinia pestis*, the word has taken on other connotations in Western cultural and literary traditions (Herzlich and Pierret 1987: 7). In the Western imagination, plague has long been envisaged as the most horrific disaster of all time. Western historical consciousness is scarred by the collective memory of the catastrophic fourteenth-century Black Death and the subsequent waves of epidemics that continued to afflict the European continent well into the eighteenth century (Carmichael 1993: 630; Park 1993: 612). As Susan Sontag (1988: 89) has eloquently argued, "plague," the disease reputed to have caused these historic epidemics, remains our most potent metaphor for utter devastation: for a cataclysm beyond belief. These images are still with us. In a recent reflection on the 1994 outbreak of pneumonic plague in India, essayist James Fenton writes that plague has left a trace in our folklore and our imaginations "as the prospect of civil life itself fatally endangered." For Fenton, "plague is not one of many epidemic diseases, but the disease of all diseases, the disease that could destroy a city, its rituals, its morality—every measure by which it reckoned its own worth" (1994: 48).

Plague, as a distinct nosological category, had no such cultural resonance in China. The contemporary name for plague, *shuyi* (literally "rat epidemic"), was not even used until the late nineteenth century.[5] Instead, plague, along with other infectious diseases manifesting in epidemics, was folded into the broad categories of *yi* (epidemics) or *dayi* (major epidemics). Localities might have their own names for disorders that occurred commonly, and in some instances local names seem to correspond to plague. In the eighteenth and nineteenth centuries, *yangzibing* in Yunnan, for example, referred to an epidemic disease that generally followed the death of rats and that caused lumps in the human body.

Disease historians rely on two distinctive features of the bubonic form of plague—rat epizootics and buboes—to identify *Yersinia pestis* infections from historical sources. The fact that humans generally contract the disease from the fleas of rodents means that descriptions of rat epizootics in the historical record may signal an outbreak of plague. The buboes that give the bubonic form its name are unusual, and mention of such symptoms in written records indicates that the disease may have been present. While suggestive of plague, reports of such phenomena cannot constitute a definitive retrospective diagnosis because the only sure way to determine whether plague is (or was) present in the human body is to conduct laboratory tests (Cunningham 1992: 209–44). Obviously, such rigid scientific criteria make it extraordinarily difficult, if not impossible, to label any past epidemic "plague." This is so even in the Western tradition, where there is some linguistic continuity in the use of the term.[6]

The post-facto identification of plague from Chinese sources is even more problematic. Not only was there no corresponding Chinese word for plague before the late nineteenth century, but Chinese observers conceptualized disease in terms very different from twentieth-century biomedicine and recorded symptoms in ways that appear vague from our modern vantage point. Serious methodological issues thus face any historian using Chinese historical records to identify a given epidemic as plague. On the one hand, we are faced with a gap between our modern sensibilities and those of pre-twentieth-century Chinese.

We are seeking something that did not exist for them—the disease biomedicine calls "plague." To name any recorded *yi* as "plague" using modern terminology is to transform it into an entity unrecognizable in the eyes, minds, and experience of those who suffered from it. On the other hand, as with plague in European history, we are unable to verify our suspicions in the microscope and must rely on descriptive evidence that falls far short of the standards imposed by the laboratory. We can thus never be certain that any particular historical episode in China was indeed plague in the modern, biomedical sense of that word.

These evidential difficulties must be kept in mind when reading the literature on the history of plague in pre-Qing China. Plague has been named as the cause of widespread epidemics in at least three distinct epochs: those that occurred at the end of the Sui and during the first two hundred years of the Tang dynasties (seventh-eighth centuries); those that affected China between the twelfth and fourteenth centuries (the Song-Yuan period); and those that accompanied the seventeenth-century Ming-Qing transition.

For the earliest period, Dr. Wu Lien-teh, a leading twentieth-century expert on the disease, cites several classical medical texts as evidence that plague has been present in China since at least the seventh century.[7] According to Wu Lien-teh (1936: 11), Chao Yuanfang's *Zhubing yuanhou zonglun* (General treatise on the etiology and symptomatology of diseases, 610 C.E.) and the *Qian jin fang* (Prescriptions worth a thousand gold, 652 C.E.) both contain descriptions of a disorder whose main symptoms were lumps on the body (*e'he*). Denis Twitchett (1979: 42, 52) also argues that at least some of the epidemics that struck China in the seventh and eighth centuries were caused by bubonic plague. Twitchett strengthens his argument with a careful reconstruction of the spatial and chronological incidence of a series of epidemics. While he acknowledges that there is no way to know whether or not plague was actually the cause of these epidemics, he notes that the timing of at least some of them was contemporaneous with what many historians believe were plague outbreaks in Central Asia and the Middle East, and he postulates a connection between the two phenomena.

Plague may have been present in China between the twelfth and fourteenth centuries. In support of this thesis, Fan Xingzhun (1986: 162–63, 241–42), a Chinese medical historian, cites numerous Song-Yuan medical texts that describe a disorder whose symptoms (the appearance of lumps, the swelling of lymphatic glands, high fevers, the coughing up of blood and phlegm) closely resemble those of various forms of plague (bubonic, septicaemic, or pneumonic). In contrast to Wu Lien-teh and Twitchett, Fan Xingzhun argues that plague did not become widespread in China until the twelfth century because the chroniclers of that time described the disease as "new."

Many historians link widespread Chinese epidemics in the Song-Yuan period to the fourteenth-century Black Death in Europe, arguing that the Black Death originated in China (Wu 1936: 47; Ziegler 1969: 15). William McNeill (1976: 143–46), for example, argues that an epidemic of bubonic plague in Hebei province in 1331 was the likely source of plague in Europe. Robert Gottfried is also persuaded that the Black Death came from China. He writes: "The first unimpeachable references appear in 1353, when chroniclers claim that two-thirds of China's population had died since 1331. Whatever the precise dates and circumstances, by the mid-fourteenth century, the Black Death had struck China" (Gottfried 1983: 35).

As John Norris (1977: 3–6) points out, the assumption that the Black Death originated in China rests on a few European chronicles and the sketchy records of epidemics found in the eighteenth-century Chinese imperial encyclopedia, the *Gujin tushu ji cheng* (Complete collection of writings and illustrations, past and present). A handful of nearly contemporaneous European sources all refer vaguely to disasters in "the East" that preceded the outbreak of plague in Europe. Sources included in the *Gujin tushu ji cheng* record a number of unspecified "epidemics" (*yi*) throughout the fourteenth century, yet there is nothing in these accounts to suggest that these epidemics were linked to the European Black Death.

The final historical period in which plague may have been widespread in China was during the Ming-Qing transition in the mid-seventeenth century. Fan Xingzhun (1986: 242–43) and another Chinese medical historian, Lee T'ao (1958: 189–90), believe that plague was responsible for the many epidemics that occurred in Zhejiang, Jiangsu, Shandong, Hubei, and Hunan in the 1640's. They cite gazetteer accounts and medical texts that they believe describe the characteristic symptoms of plague (spitting up of blood and enlarged lymph glands). Fan Xingzhun mentions that the official *Mingshi* (Ming history) and the *Dantuxian zhi* (Gazetteer of Dantu county) describe "packs of rats" that crossed rivers in large numbers prior to the outbreak of disease, and he speculates that these reports refer to the widespread death of rats preceding an epidemic of plague. Helen Dunstan (1975: 17–28) has also surveyed the seventeenth-century epidemics, and she is more skeptical than either Lee T'ao or Fan Xingzhun about whether these impressionistic descriptions of symptoms and rats refer to plague. I share Dunstan's skepticism. As the earlier discussion of plague ecology underscored, plague is a complex and varied biological phenomenon that is difficult to reconstruct using historical sources alone. Chinese chronicles provide little evidence on which to base a firm conclusion that any pre-Qing epidemic was in fact caused by *Yersinia pestis*.

Similar evidentiary dilemmas confront this study of plague in the Qing period. In local gazetteers, the primary Chinese source materials used in this book, few of the components in the disease's complicated epidemiology are recorded in the detail needed to be certain that plague was indeed present. Gazetteers typically record only the year and place where *yi* (epidemics) occurred; they seldom describe symptoms, let alone ancillary phenomena such as rat epizootics. I have used such descriptions where they exist, but in most instances no such evidence is available. Only by supplementing the historical record with knowledge drawn from modern epidemiology, medical geography, and regional analysis can an argument be made that the epidemics under discussion were caused by plague.

Fortunately for this study, there is now an extensive body of scientific and medical literature on plague published in the People's Republic of China. The Ministry of Health has given plague research high priority because the disease remains a potential public-health threat. As a result, Chinese scientists have continued to examine virtually every aspect of the disease, including the varied ecology found in China's plague reservoirs. This contemporary research adds considerably to the argument of those who find plague in China's past. Animal habitats change, of course, and plague reservoirs are not fixed for all time. Nonetheless, it is not unreasonable to assume that their existence points to a historical presence that stretches back at least two hundred years. Plague probably did afflict the Chinese in the past because the ecological conditions needed to support ongoing reservoirs of plague continue to exist in many regions of the Chinese mainland.

For the late-eighteenth-century epidemics in Yunnan, I have placed the somewhat impressionistic evidence drawn from local gazetteers into an analytical framework suggested by G. William Skinner's core-periphery regional analysis (1977a: 275–364; 1977b: 211–49; 1985: 271–92). Skinner's methodology differentiates late imperial China into eight functionally distinct macroregions defined both by physio-

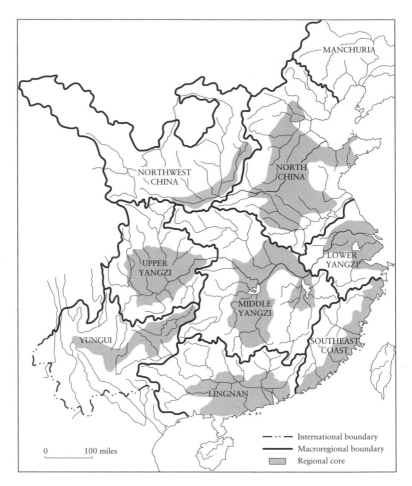

MAP 1. Macroregional systems of nineteenth-century China. Adapted from Skinner 1977b: 214–15.

graphic features and by hierarchical relationships between different types of settlements (Maps 1 and 2). Each functional macroregion is further divided into core and peripheral zones: the core river valleys and plains are distinguished by larger and denser populations, greater resource concentration, more efficient transport networks, and a higher degree of commercialization than are present in the peripheral highlands. Regional analysis is most fundamentally concerned with delineating territorially based systems of human interaction. These systems are manifested in the patterned movements of people, goods and services, money and credit, and information. The diffusion of infectious disease is another social process that can be analyzed using the regional systems perspective.

By carefully mapping the incidence of epidemics as recorded in the

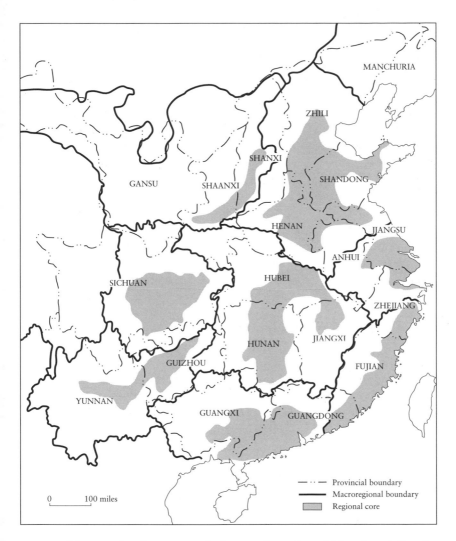

MAP 2. Macroregional systems of nineteenth-century China in relation to provinces. Adapted from Skinner 1977b: 214–15.

local gazetteers of the Yungui macroregion, I have discerned what I believe are clear spatial and temporal patterns of an epidemic that began on the western periphery of Yunnan and then moved eastward to the regional core along caravan trade routes. In the gazetteers and in official documents, there are occasional descriptions of symptoms that resemble clinical plague, and there are several references to rats dying prior to the outbreak of human epidemics. Combining these descriptive accounts with what is now known about the ecology of plague in contemporary Yunnan and the human geography of the Yungui region in the eighteenth and early nineteenth centuries, I argue that many of the epidemics recorded in the local gazetteers were most likely caused by plague.

Where possible, I also supplement Chinese-language materials with the observations of Western travelers, medical officers in the Chinese Imperial Customs Service, and United States consular officials, as well as late-nineteenth-century English and Chinese newspaper accounts. Foreigners living and traveling in China wrote about Chinese maladies using Western terminology, and they also noted the local Chinese name for the same disease. Beginning in the eighteenth century, and increasingly in the nineteenth, these observations sometimes allow Chinese terms to be matched with those concurrently in use in Western medicine. Thus Emile Rocher's firsthand observation in Yunnan in the early 1870's of a "plague-like" disease can be linked to the disease the Yunnanese termed *yangzibing* (Rocher 1879, 1: 75 and 2: 279–81; see Chapter 1).

Problems of identification are less acute for the late-nineteenth- and early-twentieth-century epidemics in southeastern China and Manchuria because foreign doctors and Western-trained Chinese physicians used biomedical concepts and terminology in their descriptions of symptoms and pathology. For the discussion of the late-nineteenth-century epidemics in the Lingnan and Southeast Coast regions (Chapters 2 and 3), I have also relied on a body of materials collected in the Chinese Academy of Medical Sciences' *Zhongguo shuyi liuxingshi* (The history of the spread of plague in China; hereafter *SYLXS*). Published in 1982, this two-volume work brings together reports on the historical incidence of plague written by local public-health departments around the country. Plague in China had been a focus of international epidemiological research since the early twentieth century, and for some areas records of plague outbreaks date back to the 1890's. After 1949, county-level sanitation and epidemic control stations (*Weisheng fangyi zhan*) were given the responsibility of documenting the history of plague in their localities. County health workers conducted oral histories, culled local gazetteers, and checked through local archival materials related to the late-nineteenth-century plague epidemics. The results of their efforts are close to eighteen hundred pages of tables, graphs, and maps documenting not only the years plague appeared but also each rural district and village thought to have been affected, and (for Fujian province) the number of cases and deaths due to plague that each village is believed to have experienced annually. I have used these reports cautiously, incorporating only those that provide adequate documentation and checking them, where possible, against other sources such as local gazetteers, Inspectorate General *Customs Medical Reports*, and United States Department of State and Public Health Service records in the National Archives (hereafter NA, USDS and NA, PHS, respectively).

In sum, while my methods and interests are primarily historical, I employ techniques and skills drawn from a number of academic and scientific disciplines, from economic geography and epidemiology to medical and cultural anthropology. I have sought to describe the dynamic relationship between the biological and social factors that were responsible for the appearance and spread of plague, as well as Chinese medical and religious representations of it. This approach allows me not only to concretely detail the history and cultural meanings of plague in Qing China but also to address broader historiographical issues related to changes in China's networks of social and economic interaction, the international politics of public health at the turn of the twentieth century, and the changing relationship between the Chinese state and society at the end of the Qing dynasty.

CHAPTER 1

Origins of Plague in Southwestern China, 1772-1898

IN CHINA TODAY, Yunnan province is celebrated for its relatively benign climate; many Chinese use the proverb "All four seasons are like spring" (*Siji ru chun*) in its praise. Yet historically the Han Chinese envisioned the southwestern frontier in far less benevolent terms. Indeed, to many who wrote about Yunnan in the past, the province was a place of pestilence and death.[1] Gazetteer compilers, for example, commonly noted that miasmas (*zhangqi*) and epidemics (*yi*) were integral parts of Yunnan's climate and history.[2] The Kangxi emperor was well aware of Yunnan's infamous *zhangqi* when he wrote the following imperial rescript in 1717:

In Yunnan, Guizhou, Guangdong, and Guangxi, there has been *zhangqi* from time immemorial. Before, when the generals attacked Yunnan, they had to leave eight hundred people in Guangxi because all had been hurt by *zhangqi*. Now, I hear that only Yuanjiang [in Yunnan] has *zhangqi*. All other places are free of it and are no different from the interior of China. (Yunnansheng lishi yanjiusuo 1984, 4: 731)

Modern epidemiological studies conducted in Yunnan suggest that the unhealthy environment described in historical records was not merely imagined. Situated on the Yungui Plateau at a latitude of 97°–106° and a longitude of 24°40'–29°15', Yunnan includes both tropical and subtropical climates within its borders. This warm climate fosters a number of animals and insects that serve as vectors for human diseases such as plague, malaria, and schistosomiasis (Tian Jingguo 1987: 141–79). The many historical references to Yunnan's *zhangqi* or *yi* suggest that before the twentieth-century advent of antibiotics and anti-malarial drugs, the southwest was often a dangerous or even deadly place.

The Eighteenth-Century Epidemics, 1772–1830

While earlier *yi*, or epidemics, are mentioned sporadically in many Yunnan gazetteers, there is a clustering of such reports for western Yunnan beginning in 1772 and lasting until about 1825 (Table 2). Some thirty years after the initial appearance of these epidemics in the west, Kunming city and its surrounding area suffered a series of epidemics beginning in 1803 and continuing until 1830 (Table 3). In 1810 a number of epidemics began to appear in Lin'an prefecture in southeastern Yunnan, and these reports lasted until 1827 (Table 4). The geographical patterning of these epidemics, as recorded in local gazetteers, suggests that they were caused by one disease that initially remained confined to the west but that eventually moved into eastern and southeastern Yunnan. One twentieth-century gazetteer for a county in southeastern Yunnan mentions that the epidemics originated in the west, an observation that lends some credence to the view that an infectious disease was moving eastward (*Shipingxian zhi* 1938, 34: 18b). If this interpretation is correct, and if these local reports reflect a provincewide epidemic that originated in western Yunnan, the question remains: What was the disease that was afflicting so many communities? Most of the reports in local gazetteers use the generic term *yi* (epidemic) and could therefore refer to any of the infectious diseases known to occur in Yunnan.

The semantic difference between the terms *zhangqi* and *yi* allows for the disqualification of certain diseases at the outset. By the beginning of the Qing period, gazetteer compilers made a clear distinction between the two. *Zhangqi* was regarded as part of an area's natural environment, and was thus mentioned in the "climate" (*qihou*) section of gazetteers. *Yi*, in contrast, were seen as events and were listed in the "disasters and omens" (*zaixiang*), "omens and strange phenomena" (*xiangyi*), or "great events" (*dashi zhi*) sections of gazetteers. Endemic malaria and schistosomiasis, chronic afflictions in many communities, were considered part of the climate of an area rather than an event (Tian Jingguo 1987: 161–64).[3] *Yi* referred to diseases that occurred episodically, came on suddenly, and affected large numbers of people at

TABLE 2
Recorded Epidemics in Western Yunnan, 1772–1825

Year	Location	Source consulted
1772–73	Heqing	*Heqingxian zhi* 1923, "zaiyi" *pian*
1776–96	Heqing	(*Xinsuan*) *Yunnan tongzhi* 1949, 10: 16
1776–96	Dali	(*Xinsuan*) *Yunnan tongzhi* 1949, 10: 16
1776–96	Langqiong	(*Xinsuan*) *Yunnan tongzhi* 1949, 10: 16
1776–96	Dengchuan	(*Xinsuan*) *Yunnan tongzhi* 1949, 10: 16
1776–96	Binchuan	(*Xinsuan*) *Yunnan tongzhi* 1949, 10: 16
1776–96	Menghua	(*Xinsuan*) *Yunnan tongzhi* 1949, 10: 16
1776–97	Zhaozhou	(*Xinsuan*) *Yunnan tongzhi* 1949, 10: 16
1776	Baiyanjing	(*Xuxiu*) *Baiyanjing zhi* 1907 [1901], 11: 13a
1776	Yaozhou	*Yanfengxian zhi* 1924, 12: 1151
1779	Lijiang	*Lijiangfu zhi* 1895, 1: 2a
1787	Dengchuan	(*Xu*) *Yunnan tongzhigao* 1901, 2: 21a
1791	Jingdong	*Jingdongxian zhigao* 1923, 2: 131
1792	Zhaozhou	Yuan Wenkui 1900 [1800], 21: 27b–29a
1792–1813	Binchuan	Hong Liangji 1877–79, 4: 3b
1796	Menghua	(*Xinsuan*) *Yunnan tongzhi* 1949, 10: 16
1798	Dengchuan	*Dengchuanzhou zhi* 1853, 5: 4a
1799	Menghua	*Menghua zhigao* 1920, 2: 2b
1799	Yongchang	*Yongchangfu zhi* 1885, 3: 8a
1799	Yuanjiang	*Yuanjiang zhigao* 1922, 6: 1
1801	Yaozhou	*Yanfengxian zhi* 1924, 12: 1152
1801	Baiyanjing	(*Xuxiu*) *Baiyanjing zhi* 1907 [1901], 11: 13a
1802	Menghua	*Menghua zhigao* 1920, 2: 2b
1803	Chuxiong	*Chuxiongxian zhi* 1910, 1: 6
1804	Dengchuan	*Dengchuanzhou zhi* 1853, 5: 4b
1804	Menghua	*Menghua zhigao* 1920, 2: 2b
1804	Yongchang	*Yongchangfu zhi* 1885, 3: 8–9
1806	Yuanjiang	(*Xu*) *Yunnan tongzhigao* 1901, 2: 22b
1816	Yongbei	(*Xuxiu*) *Yongbei zhiliting zhi* 1904, 2: 8b
1816	Yaozhou	*Yaoanxian zhi* 1948, 8: n.p.
1820	Jingdong	*Jingdongxian zhigao* 1923, 2: 132
1820	Yuanjiang	(*Xu*) *Yunnan tongzhigao* 1901, 2: 23b
1824	Jingdong	*Jingdongxian zhigao* 1923, 1: 132
1825	Dengchuan	*Dengchuanzhou zhi* 1853, 5: 5a
1825	Yunlong	*Yunlongzhou zhi* 1892, 2: 35a
1825	Langqiong	(*Xu*) *Yunnan tongzhigao* 1901, 2: 24a
1825	Yuanjiang	(*Xu*) *Yunnan tongzhigao* 1901, 2: 24a

the same time. While the recorded epidemics may have been caused by any number of infectious diseases (such as cholera, dysentery, or typhus), both modern epidemiological and historical evidence suggests that many, if not all, of the *yi* recorded for the late eighteenth and early nineteenth centuries were caused by bubonic plague.

TABLE 3

Recorded Epidemics in Eastern Yunnan, 1803–30

Year	Location	Source consulted
1803	Kunming	*Kunmingxian zhi* 1901 [1841], 8: 15a
1803	Yiliang	*Yiliangxian zhi* 1921, 1: 12
1804	Xinxing	(*Xu*) *Yunnan tongzhigao* 1901, 2: 22a
1805	Anning	(*Xu*) *Yunnan tongzhigao* 1901, 2: 22b
1805	Qujing	(*Xu*) *Yunnan tongzhigao* 1901, 2: 22b
1806	Heyang	(*Xu*) *Yunnan tongzhigao* 1901, 2: 22a
1806	Zhanyi	*Zhanyizhou zhi* 1885, 4: 80
1807	Zhanyi	(*Xu*) *Yunnan tongzhigao* 1901, 2: 22b
1808–09	Kunming	*Kunmingxian zhi* 1901 [1841], 8: 15
1809	Yiliang	*Yiliangxian zhi* 1921, 1: 12
1813	Qujing	(*Xu*) *Yunnan tongzhigao* 1901, 2: 23a
1819	Zhanyi	(*Xu*) *Yunnan tongzhigao* 1901, 2: 23b
1820	Songming	(*Xuxiu*) *Songmingzhou zhi* 1887, 2: 10a
1823	Qujing	(*Xu*) *Yunnan tongzhigao* 1901, 2: 24a
1825	Heyang	(*Xu*) *Yunnan tongzhigao* 1901, 2: 24a
1825–26	Qujing	(*Xu*) *Yunnan tongzhigao* 1901, 2: 24a
1827	Xundian	*Xundianzhou zhi* 1828, 28: 5b
1828	Anning	(*Xu*) *Yunnan tongzhigao* 1901, 2: 24a
1830	Heyang	(*Xu*) *Yunnan tongzhigao* 1901, 2: 24b

TABLE 4

Recorded Epidemics in Southeastern Yunnan, 1810–27

Year	Location	Source consulted
1810	Shiping	*Shipingxian zhi* 1938, 34: 18b–19b
1811–25	Shiping	(*Xu*) *Yunnan tongzhigao* 1901, 2: 24a
1811	Talang	*Pu'erfu zhi* 1850 [1840], 2: 10a
1812–27	Jianshui	(*Xuxiu*) *Jianshuixian zhigao* 1920, 10: 21a
1812	Mengzi	(*Xu*) *Mengzixian zhi* 1961 [1911], 12: 43a
1813	Ami	(*Xu*) *Yunnan tongzhigao* 1901, 2: 23a
1816	Mengzi	(*Xu*) *Mengzixian zhi* 1961 [1911], 12: 43a
1827	Mengzi	(*Xu*) *Mengzixian zhi* 1961 [1911], 12: 43a
1827	Jianshui	(*Xuxiu*) *Jianshuixian zhigao* 1920, 10: 21a

The Epidemiology of Plague in Contemporary Yunnan

Epidemiologists have determined that enzootic reservoirs of plague exist in parts of western Yunnan (Map 3).[4] What is called the "Western Yunnan Transverse Valley" sylvatic focus is situated in Lijiang prefecture (Zhao Yongling 1982: 257–66; Zhao Yongling and Yang Xiaodong 1983: 108–9, 113). Nestled in the foothills of the Hengduan Mountains, this prefecture has an average yearly temperature of 14.5°C, an aver-

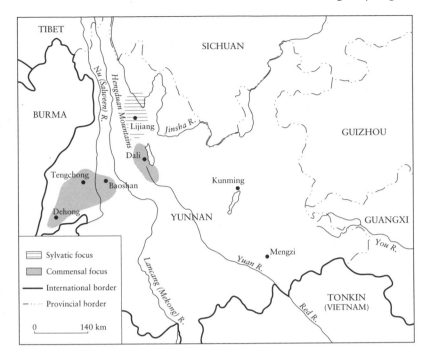

MAP 3. Sylvatic and commensal plague reservoirs in Yunnan province.

age relative humidity of 68.2 percent, and an annual precipitation of 810.6 cm. Its climate is thus hospitable to both the plague bacillus and its vectors (Tian Jingguo 1987: 145). While wild-animal plague reservoirs are found in Lijiang, commensal rat foci exist in Dali, Baoshan, and Tengchong counties and in Dehong autonomous department. Dali's climate is similar to that found in Lijiang; Baoshan, Tengchong, and Dehong lie largely west of the Nu (Salween) River in a region that is slightly hotter than Dali, with the yearly temperature averaging 19.8°C and the relative humidity averaging 76.8 percent (ibid.). These ranges also support *Yersinia pestis* and its hosts.

The known natural foci are all located in western Yunnan; eastern and southeastern Yunnan do not have the ecological conditions necessary for the formation of natural plague reservoirs. Epidemiologists believe that any plague outbreaks in the areas around the cities of Kunming or Mengzi are the result of importation of the bacteria from elsewhere. Plague epidemics in eastern Yunnan may erupt among rodent populations and last a number of years (or even decades), but without a natural reservoir to sustain continued outbreaks, the disease eventually subsides. In contrast, plague continues to be an ongoing health risk throughout much of western Yunnan.

There are ten types of mammals known to carry plague in Yunnan (*SYLXS* 1982: 760). By far the most important of these is the *Rattus flavipectus*, or yellow-chested rat. An epidemiological investigation conducted between 1952 and 1956 found specimens of this rodent in 63 out of 65 counties.[5] Subsequent studies have shown that the human disease comes almost entirely from infected *Xenopsylla cheopis* fleas that leave their *Rattus flavipectus* hosts and settle on humans following a rat epizootic.[6] The semiwild nature of this rat helps to explain the mode of transmission of plague in western Yunnan. People living near the natural plague reservoirs that exist there are in danger of coming into contact with the yellow-chested rat or any wild animals that carry plague.[7]

The bubonic form of plague is by far the most prevalent in the province: in a study done between 1950 and 1955, the bubonic form represented 91 percent out of 1,311 cases. The septicaemic form represented 7 percent, and pneumonic plague represented only 1 percent. The case-fatality rate from bubonic plague was also higher than for other forms, at 10 percent (39 out of 402 cases; *SYLXS* 1982: 770). Yunnan's mild climate allows the plague season to continue year-round. Seasonality for the human disease varies from locale to locale, but generally the plague season begins in June and July, reaches a high point in the late summer and early fall (August and September), and subsides in October (Ji Shuli 1988: 32; *SYLXS* 1982: 768).

Historical Evidence of Plague in Yunnan

The fact that enzootic foci of plague exist in western Yunnan today does not prove, of course, that particular epidemics in the past were caused by plague bacteria. As discussed in the Introduction, only when *Yersinia pestis* is microscopically seen in human tissue is such certainty possible. But in historical records of the Yunnan epidemics there are suggestive descriptions of the two distinctive features of the bubonic form of plague: rat epizootics and buboes. In reference to rat epizootics, a Chuxiong county gazetteer records rats dying in 1803, prior to the outbreak of human disease (*Chuxiongxian zhi* 1910, 1: 6). Rats died before the outbreak of human disease in southeastern Yunnan as well: a Shiping county gazetteer contains an essay on popular religious texts reputed to have been effective in warding off epidemics. It describes the 1810 epidemic in Shiping in some detail, noting that "In each family that got sick, the rats first jumped out without any reason, faltered, and fell dead in front of people. Those who saw them became sick in a very short while. Once sick, they could not be saved" (*Shipingxian zhi* 1938, 34: 18b).

Since both these accounts come from twentieth-century gazetteers, they are admittedly anachronistic. More compelling evidence of rat epizootics in western Yunnan comes from a poem entitled "Death of Rats" by Shi Daonan (1765–92), a young poet of Zhaozhou county:[8]

> Dead rats in the east,
>> Dead rats in the west!
> As if they were tigers,
>> Indeed are the people scared.
> A few days following the death of the rats,
>> Men pass away like falling walls!
> Deaths in one day are numberless,
>> The hazy sun is covered by sombre clouds.
> While three men are walking together,
>> Two drop dead within ten steps!
> People die in the night,
>> Nobody dares weep over the dead!
> The coming of the demon of pestilence
>> Suddenly makes the lamp dim,
> Then it is blown out,
>> Leaving man, ghost, and corpse in the dark room.
> The crows caw incessantly,
>> The dogs howl bitterly!
> Man and ghost are as one,
>> While the spirit is taken for a human being!
> The land is filled with human bones,
>> There in the fields are crops,
> To be reaped by none;
>> And the officials collect no tax!
> I hope to ride on a fairy dragon
>> To see the God and Goddess in heaven,
> Begging them to spread heavenly milk,
>> And make the dead come to life again.

This poem is part of a longer one, entitled "Tian yu ji," mentioned by Hong Liangji (Hong Beijiang, 1736–1809) in his collected works (1877–79, 4: 3b).[9] In discussing Shi Daonan's poetry, Hong Liangji describes the "strange rats" of Zhaozhou who came out of the ground in the daytime, spit up blood, and fell dead. People "breathing the vapor of the dead rats" quickly became ill and died.

A memorial written in 1814 by the Yunnan provincial education commissioner (*xuezheng*), Gu Chun (Gu Xihan, 1790–1860), provides further contemporaneous evidence that the disease spreading throughout the province between 1772 and 1830 was most likely bubonic plague.[10] Gu Chun describes symptoms characteristic of the bubonic form of plague: spitting up of blood and buboes on the bodies of plague victims. Such a detailed description of symptoms is highly unusual in an official report; indeed, it is the only such description I have found in memorials reporting outbreaks of epidemic disease. This suggests that Gu Chun found the symptoms particularly noteworthy. He underscores the eastward progression of the disease, mentioning that the area around Jianshui county (in Lin'an prefecture) was not affected until 1810 or so, but that other parts of the province had been experiencing the same disease, *yangzibing*, for more than ten years.[11] He mentions that doctors in the Lin'an area did not recognize the disease: this is significant because it suggests that plague was new to Lin'an. Finally, he describes a great number of deaths during the epidemic and says that there was no known medicine for treating those afflicted. Taken together with the geographical pattern of epidemics recorded in gazetteers, scattered references to rat epizootics, and Shi Daonan's poetic description, Gu Chun's memorial suggests that Yunnan was indeed experiencing an outbreak of bubonic plague at the turn of the nineteenth century.

Regional Economic Change and the Spread of Plague

Chinese epidemiologists have worked from the hypothesis that the contemporary existence of a natural plague reservoir in the western part of Yunnan province implies a historical existence there as well (Ji Shuli 1988: 15–16). This assumes continuity in the natural environment over the past two hundred years, a presumption that requires further research in the areas of climatic and ecological change. Leaving aside the difficult and perhaps unanswerable question of when the western Yunnan plague reservoir first formed, it is still possible to address the problem of why plague erupted on such a large scale in Yunnan in the late eighteenth century. This requires an analysis of changes in the economy of the Yungui macroregion, of which Yunnan is a part.[12]

The Yungui region is on a high plateau containing eight mountain ranges and hundreds of deep valleys cut by fast-moving and generally nonnavigable rivers (J. Lee 1993: 91). Preindustrial transport in the region had to move overland, and, even then, the steep mountain roads between isolated settlements limited trade to commodities that could be carried by human porters or mule train. These transportation difficulties made urban and economic development in the southwest lag far behind the eastern coastal provinces, where travel and shipping were much easier (Naquin and Rawski 1987: 205).

Yungui did not begin to change from an undeveloped frontier into a dynamic regional economy until the Ming-Qing period. The region experienced an initial burst of economic and demographic expansion in the fifteenth century, but this growth was interrupted by the warfare of the Ming-Qing transition in the mid-seventeenth century (J. Lee 1982a: 720). With the defeat of the Rebellion of the Three Feudatories in 1681, the southwest began its takeoff. Around 1700 the Yungui region entered an economic upswing that continued into the first decades of the nineteenth century. By the 1830's this regional growth had slowed considerably, but for more than a century the southwest experienced explosive population increases, rapid urban development, and expanded intraregional and interregional trade. These changes in the regional economy of Yungui greatly facilitated the spread of bubonic plague throughout Yunnan.

Yunnan's Economic and Demographic Growth, 1700–1800.　As James Lee (1993: 257–96) has demonstrated, the eighteenth-century transformation of the Yungui region was primarily a consequence of governmental support for southwestern copper mining. Although provincial authorities began regulating the Yunnan copper industry in 1705, mining intensified after 1723, when the Tokugawa regime in Japan ordered that all exports of Japanese copper to China be stopped. With the central Qing government providing supervision, incentives, and subsidies, Chinese merchant-entrepreneurs revived old mines, opened new ones, and vastly increased copper production in the southwest. By the end of the eighteenth century, Yunnan mines had produced more than half a million metric tons of copper—approximately one-fifth of total world production (ibid.: 261).

The development of the Yunnan mining industry spurred Han Chinese immigration into the province and resulted in substantial population growth. Between 1750 and 1800, more than three hundred thousand miners from Sichuan, Jiangxi, and Hunan (and some from

Guangdong, Hubei, and Shaanxi) poured into Yunnan (J. Lee 1982b: 299). What had previously been rural hinterland or wilderness was soon filled with bustling mining camps.[13] Immigrant merchants followed, drawn by the economic opportunities of providing services to the mining population. A labor class emerged to work in manufacturing and transport. In 1775 the registered population of Yunnan was over three million people and the average annual rate of growth was approximately seven per thousand, a rate that James Lee estimates to be consistent with the national average for the same time period. By his calculations, Yunnan's average annual rate of population growth began to rise after 1775, reaching ten per thousand by 1785 and hitting a very high twenty per thousand by 1795, a rate that did not slow until after 1811 (1982a: 731).

The large influx of Han immigrants also altered settlement patterns in the region. Miners had to be near mineral deposits, of course, and their rough camps eventually grew into small towns. As merchants and transport workers arrived, Yunnan was transformed from a predominantly rural region to an increasingly urban one. Before 1750, only the town of Jianshui had reached a population of 50,000 (J. Lee 1982b: 300–301). Dali and Kunming had populations of about 30,000. Two towns along the major trade routes with Burma, Simao and Tengyue, barely reached 5,000. James Lee has estimated that, before 1750, the aggregate urban population of the Yungui macroregion was about 5 percent of the total southwest population, the lowest proportion of urban to rural population for any region in China (ibid.). By 1830, however, the total urban population had grown to about 10 percent of the entire population, a very high percentage in China at the time.

The expansion of urban settlements within the region brought with it an increase in intraregional trade. Due to the difficulties of overland transport in Yunnan, the state played a central role in organizing the production and transport of grain and salt to emergent urban centers. It encouraged the opening of new agricultural regions in the far west of the province, on the border near Burma, and it helped develop and maintain commercial infrastructure (J. Lee 1982a: 741; 1993: 91–94). Paved roads and bridges were built or repaired with government sponsorship.[14] The need to ship copper ore and agricultural products, such as tea, beyond provincial borders also stimulated interregional trade.

Long-distance traders traveled through the province along several major roads (Map 4).[15] A number of routes linked Kunming, the provin-

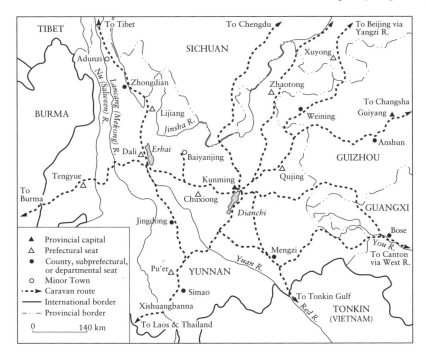

MAP 4. Caravan trade routes in Yunnan province, ca. 1800.

cial capital of Yunnan, to central and northern China: copper ore and other minerals were transported to Beijing along the Yangzi River via a route that ran northward from Kunming to Qujing prefecture, into Guizhou province (through Weining) and Sichuan (via Xuyong), and finally down the river (Luzhou–Hankou–Yizheng–Yangzhou–[Grand Canal]–Tongzhou–Beijing). Although this path had been used as an official and commercial route during the Tang dynasty, it was virtually abandoned during the Ming period and was only reopened under the Qing (Lombard-Salmon 1972: 94; Sun 1971). An alternate way to the Yangzi (via Xuzhou [Yibin] and Chongqing) passed first through the town of Zhaotong (Carné 1982 [1872]: 333–39; Hosie 1890: 55–66). Kunming was linked to Changsha via Guiyang along a route that was in use as early as the third century (Kunming–Qujing–Guiyang–Zhenzhou [Yuanling]–Changsha; see Lombard-Salmon 1972: 94). Yet another route led northward from Kunming to Chengdu (J. Lee 1993: 93).

Two routes led from southeastern Yunnan to Canton, both of which came to be used extensively during the nineteenth century. The first was along the Yuan River, which turns south from Mengzi and flows through Vietnam (where it is called the Red River) into the Tonkin Gulf. From Vietnam, sailing vessels carried goods to southern Chinese ports, including Canton. The second followed the You River and passed through the towns of Bose and Nanning in Guangxi before connecting with the West (Xi) River in Guangdong. This route was first developed by the Qing in 1729, and it was destined to become a major artery between Yunnan and the southeast littoral in the last century of Qing rule (J. Lee 1993: 94, 335; see Chapter 2).

The trade routes between Yunnan and Southeast Asian states date back to the eight and ninth centuries (Forbes 1987: 3). During the Tang dynasty, a road passed from Chongqing across the Jinsha (Golden Sand) River to Dali prefecture and from there to Burma. Although the northern part of this route had been largely abandoned by the time the Manchus conquered China, the section between Dali and Burma was still being used during the Qing period. Burmese cotton was sent up the Irrawaddy River in large boats as far as Mandalay and then traded with Yunnanese traders at Madah or at Bhamao. From there it was carried overland by mule train along a route that ran from the frontier town of Tengyue in the west to Dali and then on to Kunming (Shi Fan 1891b, 13: 7913–14; T'ien 1982: 24). Two caravan routes also ran southward from Simao to northern Thailand, one passing through Laos, the other through Burma (Forbes 1987: 45). The Yunnan-Tibetan tea trade was of similar antiquity, dating back possibly to the eighth century. The first written records of the trade date to 1398. Pu'er tea, grown in Xishuangbanna on the Yunnan-Lao border, was processed at Pu'er and then transported by mule caravan to the prefectural town of Lijiang, where it was sold to wholesalers (Hill 1989: 324–25). From there, merchants from Lijiang transported the tea to Tibet, passing through Zhongdian and Adunzi on their way.[16]

Yunnan's distant location and internal topography imposed constraints on the amount of interregional and intraregional trade conducted in the province, even during the boom of the eighteenth and early nineteenth centuries. The fact that only overland transport was possible meant that travel times were slower than in regions of China where navigable waterways were plentiful (J. Lee 1993: 95, 331–37). Nonetheless, commodities such as Pu'er tea, salt, and copper ore commanded a high enough price to make the long-distance haul worth the trouble.[17] As James Lee (ibid.: 102) has pointed out, the eighteenth-century Qing state invested heavily in improving communications and transportation in the southwest, and as a result roads were slightly more accessible to travelers than they had been earlier. Increases in population, the development of towns, and state investment in mining and transportation all stimulated trade to such an extent that the number of caravans moving along Yunnan's trade corridors undoubtedly increased from 1700 on.

Commercial Expansion and the Spread of Plague, 1772–1830. Where and how Yunnan was first infected with plague is a question that is unresolvable, but it seems likely that the origins of the late-eighteenth-century epidemic lie in the enzootic plague foci of western China. The fact that Jianchuan county in Lijiang prefecture now forms a natural reservoir for the disease has led some Chinese epidemiologists to hypothesize that plague was already enzootic there before the eighteenth century. Others believe that the plague bacillus was imported into the province from Burma or Tibet (Ji Shuli 1988: 15–16).[18] Both hypotheses seem tenable. The central point here is that the eighteenth-century intensification of long-distance trade through wilderness areas of Lijiang prefecture facilitated the spread of plague to the increasingly more populated areas of Yunnan.

In the late eighteenth century, Lijiang prefecture was regionally peripheral in the sense that it had low population densities (six people per square kilometer in 1795, and seven in 1805) relative to other prefectures in the province (J. Lee 1982a: 730). However, the town of Lijiang was the major wholesaling center for the Pu'er-Tibetan tea trade. Lijiang merchants held a monopoly on the trade by virtue of a state licensing system (R. Lee 1979: 50). The Pu'er-Tibetan tea trade was particularly active during the period of Qing expansion along the Sino-Tibetan border (1701–95), when strong military control of the frontier region allowed traders to move back and forth without fear of tribal raids. As more and more traders passed through Lijiang prefecture, they either inadvertently brought plague from Tibet into Yunnan along the Tibetan-Lijiang road, or they passed through an area where plague was already enzootic. Either way, they came into contact with plague-infected fleas and eventually carried them back to the towns and cities in the regional core.

Closer examination of the geographical pattern of epidemics listed in Tables 2, 3, and 4 supports this hypothesis. In about 1772 a series

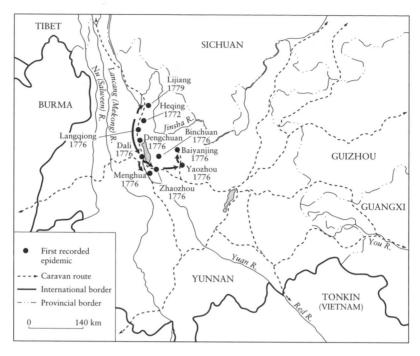

MAP 5. Recorded epidemics in Yunnan, 1772–79.

of epidemics began to appear in settlements lying near or along the Yunnan-Tibetan route (Map 5). The first record of what may have been a plague outbreak is the 1772 epidemic recorded in Heqing (*Heqingxian zhi* 1923: "zaiyi" *pian*). Assuming that the disease causing this epidemic was indeed plague, it is possible to trace its spread further along the route used to transport Pu'er tea from Yunnan to Tibet. By 1776 epidemics were prevalent not only in Heqing but also in most of the localities around Dali, including Zhaozhou, Langqiong, Dengchuan, and Binchuan ([*Xinsuan*] *Yunnan tongzhi* 1949, 10: 16). Epidemics also appeared in 1776 in the area of Menghua, an entrepôt along the tea route, in the area around the saltwells at Baiyanjing, and in Yaozhou, a town on the road leading to the saltwells (ibid. 10: 16; [*Xuxiu*] *Baiyanjing zhi* 1907 [1901], 11: 13a; *Yanfengxian zhi* 1924, 12: 1151). Three years later, in 1779, an epidemic occurred in Lijiang prefecture (*Lijiangfu zhi* 1895, 1: 2a).

As Map 6 shows, Jingdong had an epidemic outbreak in 1791

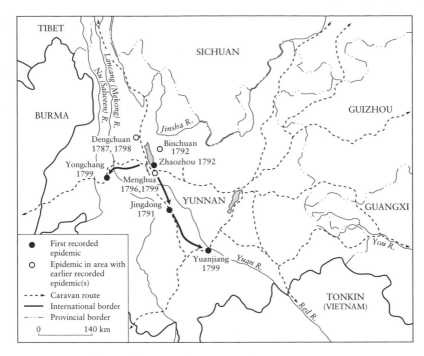

MAP 6. Recorded epidemics in Yunnan, 1787–99.

(*Jingdongxian zhigao* 1923, 2: 131). Yuanjiang autonomous department, downriver from Jingdong, was stricken in 1799, and Yongchang prefecture, to the west of Dali on the road to Burma, had an outbreak in the same year (*Yongchangfu zhi* 1885, 3: 8a; *Yuanjiang zhigao* 1922, 6: 1). Other communities, such as Dengchuan, Binchuan, and Zhaozhou, again experienced epidemics during the 1790's.

No information is available on mortality due to these epidemics for this early period, but the western region around Dali appears to have been hit hard. In Dengchuan department, on the northern tip of Er'hai Lake, more than "ten thousand" people supposedly died in the 1787 epidemic ([*Xu*] *Yunnan tongzhigao* 1901, 2: 21a). Sometime around 1800, the village of Yangtangli in Dengchuan department experienced an epidemic so devastating that it had not recovered fifty years later. Reportedly, "nine out of ten" houses were left empty by disease (*Dengchuanzhou zhi* 1853, 3: 11b). While these figures are largely formulaic, they nonetheless suggest that the epidemics around Dali caused many deaths. Shi Daonan's poem, quoted earlier, evokes images of great suffering and loss of life, and we know that he, his mother, and other relatives died in the 1792 outbreak in Zhaozhou (Yuan Wenkui 1900 [1800], 21: 27b).

From the initial recorded outbreak in 1772 until the late 1790's, these epidemics remained largely confined to western Yunnan. During this same period of time (1775–95), as has already been made clear, the provincial population was growing very rapidly, a development that spurred even greater intraregional commerce. Increased movement of trade caravans between eastern and western Yunnan probably allowed infected rats or their fleas to be carried along the main route linking Dali to Kunming. Indeed, as indicated in Table 3 and Map 7, widespread epidemics began to break out in the area around Kunming in 1803, and shortly thereafter in jurisdictions situated along Yunnan's eastern highways: Yiliang was affected in 1803, Qujing in 1805, and Zhanyi in 1806 (*Kunmingxian zhi* 1901 [1841], 8: 15a; [*Xu*] *Yunnan tongzhigao* 1901, 2: 22b; *Yiliangxian zhi* 1921, 1: 12; *Zhanyizhou zhi* 1885, 4: 80). Epidemics also appeared in communities on the plain surrounding Kunming: Xinxing in 1804, Anning in 1805, and Heyang in 1806 ([*Xu*] *Yunnan tongzhigao* 1901, 2: 22a).

The Kunming region experienced repeated epidemics for some years after the initial recorded outbreak in 1803. At the same time, the disease spread farther southward along the roads leading to Jianshui (in Lin'an prefecture; see Table 4 and Map 8). The population in the southeastern part of the province had grown significantly in the late eighteenth century after the Gejiu tin mines were opened (*Mengzixian zhi* 1797 [1791], 3: 45a). Again, such population growth must have stimulated greater movement between Jianshui and Kunming, a development that probably accounts for the eventual spread of plague to the southeastern subregion. Shiping had periodic epidemics beginning in 1810 and lasting until 1825; Talang in 1811; Jianshui and Mengzi in 1812; and Ami in 1813 (*Pu'erfu zhi* 1850 [1840], 2: 10a; *Shipingxian zhi* 1938, 34: 18b–19b; [*Xu*] *Mengzixian zhi* 1961 [1911], 12: 43a; [*Xu*] *Yunnan tongzhigao* 1901, 2: 23a; [*Xuxiu*] *Jianshuixian zhigao* 1920, 10: 21a). Many of these areas continued to experience epidemics into the 1820's.[19]

There are few narrative descriptions of plague's impact on eastern and southeastern Yunnan. Gu Chun, the education commissioner mentioned earlier, notes in his memorial that "a hundred thousand" (i.e., a very great number) died from *yangzibing* in the Lin'an area, and

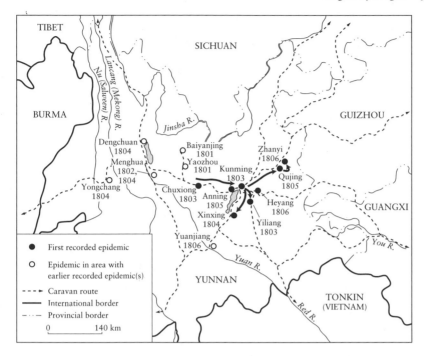

MAP 7. Recorded epidemics in Yunnan, 1801–7.

a county gazetteer describes how, during the 1811 epidemic in Shiping, "Those seen in the morning were dead by evening. In the space of one or two days, several people in the same family were all dead" (*Shipingxian zhi* 1938, 34: 18b–19b). Fewer jurisdictions were affected for a shorter period of time in eastern Yunnan than in western Yunnan, and so mortality was probably lower in the area around Kunming and Lin'an than it was in communities of the Dali region.

Although epidemics continued to be recorded in Yunnan's local gazetteers between 1815 and 1830 (Map 9), such reports drop off after 1825, and between the 1830's and the early 1850's only a handful of gazetteers, mostly those situated in western-central Yunnan, contain references to epidemics (Table 5 and Map 10). The 1910 Chuxiong county gazetteer reports that an epidemic of plague (*shuyi*) broke out in Chuxiong between 1844 and 1845 (*Chuxiongxian zhi* [1910], 1: 6). Menghua, to the west of Chuxiong, reportedly had *yi* between 1846

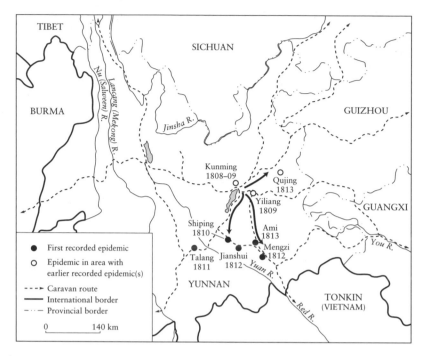

MAP 8. Recorded epidemics in eastern Yunnan, 1808–13.

and 1847 (*Menghua zhigao* 1920, 2: 3a). Dali appears to have had an epidemic in 1851, and Heyang had one in 1852 (*Dalixian zhigao* 1917, 3: 8a; *Yunnan tongzhi* 1894: n.p.).

The relative paucity of recorded epidemics in Yunnan between 1830 and 1850 may be the consequence of a slowdown in the amount of traffic moving along Yunnan's various trade routes following the economic slump that hit the Yungui region in the first half of the nineteenth century. The Yunnan copper industry that had spurred the eighteenth-century upswing in the regional economy was now a central factor in the region's decline. By the 1760's many copper deposits were already mined out; only the infusion of massive state subsidies allowed productivity to remain high for several more decades (J. Lee 1993: 279–82). As the ore continued to be depleted in the 1780's and 1790's, rising copper prices gradually reduced demand. By the end of the eighteenth century, the state was forced to halt its copper mining subventions altogether, a move that precipitated the rapid clo-

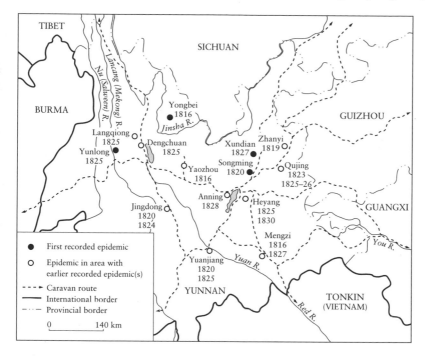

MAP 9. Recorded epidemics in Yunnan, 1815–30.

sure of about a quarter of Yunnan's mines and eventually pushed the province into a recession (ibid.: 285; Sun 1968: 841).

Declining economic opportunities in the mines discouraged further immigration into the province, a phenomenon reflected in slowing population growth rates after 1811. Although James Lee (1982a: 731) estimates that between 1775 and 1825 the average annual rate of Yunnan's population growth was double the rate of increase in China's registered population at large, by 1845 growth rates of the provincial population had slowed to an average annual rate *lower* than the national average of seven per thousand. In the early part of the nineteenth century, opium was just beginning to emerge as Yunnan's major cash crop; it was not a major impetus to trade before 1840 (see Chapter 2). Slowdowns in the mining industry and in immigration almost certainly depressed commerce and trade in the province for a time, and consequently the diffusion of plague slowed as well.

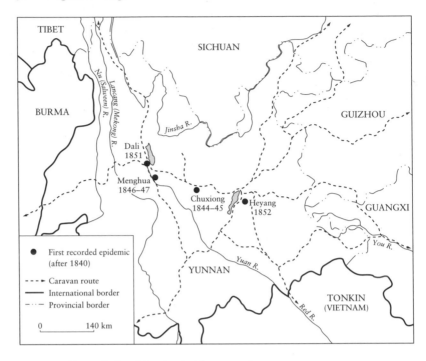

MAP 10. Recorded epidemics in Yunnan, 1844–52.

TABLE 5
Recorded Epidemics in Yunnan, 1844–52

Year	Location	Source consulted
1844–45	Chuxiong	*Chuxiongxian zhi* 1910, 1: 6
1846–47	Menghua	*Menghua zhigao* 1920, 2: 3a
1851	Dali	*Dalixian zhigao* 1917, 3: 8a
1852	Heyang	*Yunnan tongzhi* 1894: n.p.

The Nineteenth-Century Epidemics, 1854–98

Although Yunnan's economic growth faltered in the first half of the nineteenth century, the province was clearly a different place than it had been some fifty years earlier. By the middle of the nineteenth century, Yunnan was both more populated and more highly integrated into long-distance trading networks than it had been in 1800.

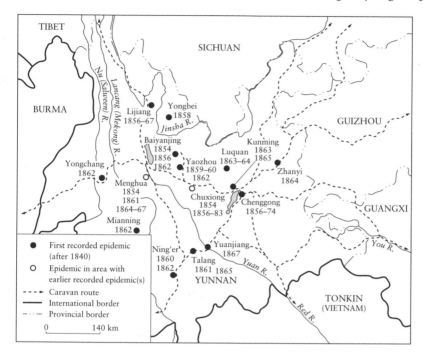

MAP 11. Recorded epidemics in Yunnan, 1854–70.

There were now many more people in the province: the registered population in 1800 had been 4,455,309, but in 1850 it was 7,375,503 (J. Lee 1982a: 722–23). Given this more densely populated and more highly integrated commercial environment, plague could spread more quickly and more extensively through the human population if it again appeared in the province. Indeed, a second wave of epidemics did emerge in Yunnan in the middle of the nineteenth century, beginning in the early 1850's and lasting several decades (Maps 11 and 12).[20] Whereas the late-eighteenth- and early-nineteenth-century epidemics were largely the consequence of an upsurge in commercial traffic, those of the mid-nineteenth century were more likely precipitated by troop movements and refugee migrations during the violent conflict that engulfed Yunnan for the seventeen years from 1856 and 1873 — namely, the Muslim Rebellion.

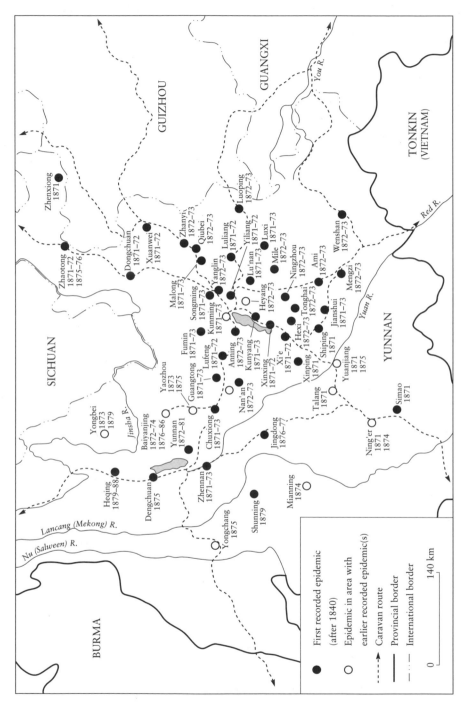

MAP 12. Recorded epidemics in Yunnan, 1871–79.

*The Muslim Rebellion and the Reemergence
of Plague, 1856–73*

The Muslim Rebellion was sparked by disputes in 1854 between Han
and Muslim miners in Chuxiong prefecture (Wang Xuhuai 1968; Wei
1974; and Wright 1957: 113–17). What began as a localized argument
eventually erupted into large-scale violence. On May 19, 1856, more
than a thousand Muslims were massacred in Kunming and the surrounding countryside. The massacre set off retaliatory killing throughout the province. Under the leadership of Du Wenxiu, Muslims in the
western half of Yunnan established a separatist government in the city
of Dali. A second rebel force under Ma Rulong kept military pressure
on the Qing forces in central and eastern Yunnan until 1862, when
Ma Rulong transferred his loyalty to the Qing government. Between
1862 and 1868 a truce was declared, and for seven years Yunnan experienced relative peace. Then Ma Rulong, together with Cen Yuying,
carried out a relentless campaign to force the Dali Muslims to surren-
der. From 1868 to 1872 the area between Kunming and Dali was the
scene of constant troop movement and siege warfare. Qing forces recovered the Muslim bases in southern, eastern, and central Yunnan by
1870. In 1872 loyalist soldiers placed the Muslim stronghold of Dali
under siege, and the city was finally captured in January 1873. Du
Wenxiu committed suicide, and the Qing army destroyed the city. The
government had to take three other western towns before the rebellion was put down completely in June 1873.

The Muslim Rebellion created enormous disruption in Yunnan and
seemingly brought population growth there to a halt. According to
the Yunnan provincial gazetteer, in 1830 the registered population of
the province was 6,553,108 ([*Xu*] *Yunnan tongzhigao* 1901, 35: 3b). In
1850 it was 7,375,503, and in 1855 it was 7,522,000. But by 1884 the
registered population had dropped to only 2,982,664.[21] This drop was
undoubtedly due to mortality from military violence, to famine, and
to emigration from the province. Epidemic diseases, including plague,
also devastated the population. A statement from a Menghua gazetteer sums up the multiple catastrophes many communities suffered:
"Three in ten died in the war, one in ten died from epidemics, and one
or two in ten fled. Only four or five out of ten are left" (*Menghua xianxiang tuzhi*, Guangxu edition, *hukou* [population] section).

Given the degree of chaos in Yunnan and the prevalence of famine
during these years, the population no doubt suffered from many differ-

ent infections, including the "famine fevers" of typhus and dysentery. Cholera may have been present as well. But historical evidence again suggests that many of the epidemics, if not the majority of them, were caused by bubonic plague. Several gazetteer accounts describe how *yangzibing*—the same disease that had first appeared at the turn of the century—reappeared during the Muslim Rebellion (*Xinan biancheng Mianning wuzhang* 1937, 3: 81; *Yaoanxian zhi* 1948, 66: 12a). Foreign accounts of conditions in Yunnan during and immediately after the war also tell of plague in the province. A French expedition led by Doudart de Lagrée traveled through Yunnan in the winter of 1867–68; as they moved from Dongchuan to Dali, they heard that rats had been found dead in large numbers in an opium den (Carné 1982 [1872]: 309–10). The French believed this was a testament to the overpowering fumes of opium, but it was more likely the result of a rat-plague epizootic.

Shortly after the rebellion had been suppressed in eastern Yunnan (1871–73), a French member of the Chinese Imperial Customs Service, Emile Rocher, made an extensive tour of pacified areas of the province. His notes on the virulent epidemics he witnessed leave little doubt that Yunnan was again experiencing large-scale outbreaks of bubonic plague (Rocher 1879, 2: 279–81).[22] Rocher observed what he believed were two separate epidemics, one beginning in Pu'er prefecture (in southwestern Yunnan) in 1871, spreading as far north as Zhaotong prefecture (in the northeast), and ending in Heiyan (in western-central Yunnan) in 1872 (ibid.: map folder). Rocher reported that the second epidemic began in the area around Kunming in 1872 and spread throughout much of east and southeastern Yunnan in 1873, and he noted that outbreaks of human disease were invariably preceded by the death of rats. The first sign of the disease in humans was a fever that became very high within a few hours. Lumps appeared in the lymph nodes, usually in the armpits, the groin, or the neck. Often the patient lost consciousness or slipped into delirium. If the lumps ruptured, recovery was possible; otherwise, death was virtually certain. Rocher estimated that in areas where the epidemic was very light, about 4 percent of the population fell ill. In some areas entire families died and the population was almost wiped out.[23]

The Differential Impact of Plague on Yunnan's Subregions

The social and economic effects both of the Muslim Rebellion and of repeated plague epidemics were felt most acutely in the western part

TABLE 6
Recorded Epidemics in Western Yunnan, 1854–96

Year	Location	Source consulted
1854	Menghua	*Menghua zhigao* 1920, 2: 3b
1856–67	Lijiang	*Lijiangfu zhi* 1895, 1: 2b
1858	Yongbei	(*Xuxiu*) *Yongbei zhiliting zhi* 1904, 2: 9a
1861	Menghua	*Menghua zhigao* 1920, 2: 3b
1862	Mianning	*Mianningxian zhi* 1945, n.p.
1862	Yongchang	*Yongchangfu zhi* 1885, 28: 27
1864–67	Menghua	*Menghua zhigao* 1920, 2: 3b
1873	Yongbei	(*Xuxiu*) *Yongbei zhiliting zhi* 1904, 2: 9b
1874	Mianning	*Mianningxian zhi* 1945, n.p.
1875	Dengchuan	*Yunnan tongzhi* 1894, n.p.
1875	Yongchang	*Yongchangfu zhi* 1885, 3: 9b
1879	Shunning	(*Xu*) *Yunnan tongzhigao* 1901, 2: 23a
1879	Yongbei	(*Xuxiu*) *Yongbei zhiliting zhi* 1904, 2: 10a
1879–88	Heqing	*Heqingzhou zhi* 1894, 2: 4b
1881	Yongbei	(*Xuxiu*) *Yongbei zhiliting zhi* 1904, 2: 10b
1889–94	Yongbei	(*Xuxiu*) *Yongbei zhiliting zhi* 1904, 2: 10b
1890	Lijiang	*Lijiangfu zhi* 1895, 1: 2b
1890	Menghua	*Menghua zhigao* 1920, 2: 3b
1891	Yongbei	(*Xuxiu*) *Yongbei zhiliting zhi* 1904, 2: 10a
1892	Dengchuan	(*Xinsuan*) *Yunnan tongzhi* 1949, 10: 16
1894	Mianning	*Kunmingxian zhi* 1901 [1841], 8: 15b
1896	Langqiong	*Langqiongxian zhilue* 1903, 1: 5b

of Yunnan. When imperial soldiers retook the area, they exacted harsh retribution against the Dali rebels. Dali city was subjected to a six-month siege in 1872–73, and when it was finally captured, after three days of murder and arson, an estimated fifty thousand were dead or missing (Wright 1957: 117). Recovery after the war was extremely slow. When William Gill (1883: 249) passed through Dali in September 1877, the city was still devastated. In April 1883, Alexander Hosie saw only "two good streets, the rest of the city was in ruins" (1890: 138).

The greatest damage in western Yunnan was sustained by towns along the road between Kunming and Dali, and on the plain west of Er'hai Lake. Death and emigration had greatly reduced the population of settlements on the Dali Plain: before the rebellion the largest villages had some seven to eight hundred families, but in 1877 they had only two to three hundred (Gill 1883: 250).[24] The towns along the highway to Kunming lay in ruins: in 1883 only Zhaozhou showed any signs of recovery. Zhennan, Chuxiong, Guangtong, Lufeng, and Anning were all in "a very dilapidated condition. In most of them the walls, which were breached, had not been repaired; nor within the walls was there

TABLE 7
Recorded Epidemics in Western-Central Yunnan, 1854–83

Year	Location	Source consulted
1854	Baiyanjing	(*Xuxiu*) *Baiyanjing zhi* 1907 [1901], 11: 14a–14b
1854	Chuxiong	*Chuxiongxian zhi* 1910, 1: 6
1856	Baiyanjing	(*Xuxiu*) *Baiyanjing zhi* 1907 [1901], 1: 14a–14b
1856–83	Chuxiong	*Chuxiongxian zhi* 1910, 1: 6
1859–60	Yaozhou	*Yaozhou zhi* 1885, 11: 12a
1862	Yaozhou	*Yanfengxian zhi* 1924, 12: 1154
1862	Baiyanjing	(*Xuxiu*) *Baiyanjing zhi* 1907 [1901], 11: 14b
1871–72	Lufeng	Rocher 1879: map folder
1871–72	Guangtong	Rocher 1879: map folder
1871–72	Chuxiong	Rocher 1879: map folder
1871–72	Zhennan	Rocher 1879: map folder
1872–73	Nan'an	Rocher 1879: map folder
1872–73	Chuxiong	Rocher 1879: map folder
1872–73	Guangtong	Rocher 1879: map folder
1872–73	Zhennan	Rocher 1879: map folder
1872–74	Baiyanjing	(*Xuxiu*) *Baiyanjing zhi* 1907 [1901], 11: 15a
1872–81	Yunnan	*Yunnanxian zhi* 1890, 1: 7
1873	Yaozhou	*Yanfengxian zhi* 1924, 12: 1154
1875	Yaozhou	*Yaozhou zhi* 1885, 11: 12b
1876–86	Baiyanjing	(*Xuxiu*) *Baiyanjing zhi* 1907 [1901], 11: 15a
1878–83	Yaozhou	*Yaozhou zhi* 1885, 11: 13a

any marked indication of returning prosperity" (Hosie 1890: 140). Towns along the roads west of Dali also suffered severely: Yongping, for example, had been almost totally destroyed (Gill 1883: 263).

Prefectures and counties along the western trade routes were hard hit by disease as well. Between 1854—when localized violence first broke out in Yunnan—and 1862, epidemics appeared in Menghua, Lijiang, Mianning, Yongbei, and Yongchang (*Lijiangfu zhi* 1895, 1: 2b; *Menghua zhigao* 1920, 2: 3b; *Mianningxian zhi* 1945: n.p.; [*Xuxiu*] *Yongbei zhiliting zhi* 1904, 2: 9a; *Yongchangfu zhi* 1885, 28: 27). (See Table 6.) Yaozhou and Chuxiong, on the sideroad to the Baiyanjing saltwells, as well as other counties in western-central Yunnan, suffered repeated epidemics both right before, during, and after the war years (*Chuxiongxian zhi* 1910, 1: 6; [*Xuxiu*] *Baiyanjing zhi* 1907 [1901], 11: 14b; *Yaozhou zhi* 1885, 11: 12a). (See Table 7.)

Both gazetteer accounts and foreign observations describe the ravages of these epidemics. In Yaozhou county, people reportedly died "like weeds" following an epidemic (*Yaoanxian zhi* 1948, 66: 12a). The town of Mianning (in Shunning prefecture) "became completely empty" as a result of the epidemics that occurred for some thirteen years after the rebellion (*Xinan biancheng Mianning wuzhang* 1937, 3: 81; see also *Dalixian zhigao* 1917, 3: 8a). In the valley around Yongbei, "A deadly plague annually sweeps down the valley and mows down its inhabitants" (Hosie 1890: 127). Archibald Colquhoun described the effects of plague on the town of Jingdong as follows:

This scene of ruin, in such a peaceful valley, bespeaking peaceful prosperity, if ever a scene did, culminated in Ching-tung [Jingdong]. Here we found, not the city which we had expected—from its position in the grand valley, half-way between the south and Tali [Dali]—but a paltry village. If the place today is really only a village of some 500 houses, it shows signs—evident to the eye, without any telling,—that it has a very different past history. The half-ruined outer walls, yamens, and gateways and buildings of various sorts, both in the inner town and through the ruined suburbs, bespoke of past prosperity. The estimate given me by the Prefect that it has dwindled down from 5,000 houses to 500, and these of small importance, seems quite reasonable. According to him, the plain is stricken by the terrible scourge, the Yunnan plague . . . if the plague were stamped out, the city and valley would rapidly recover, there can be no doubt. (Colquhoun 1883, 2: 137)

When William Gill passed along the road from Dali to Burma, he found that the town of Pupiao near Yongchang had just suffered an intense epidemic of plague:

The main road . . . passes through the plain of Fu-Piau [Pupiao] which had been entirely depopulated by an extraordinary disease, of which the symptoms were like those of the plague and which had, during the months of August and September, carried off upwards of a thousand people. Our informant added that there was no one left except a few poverty-stricken wretches, who could not afford to move. A traveller who was stopping at the same inn with us at Yung-Ch'ang [Yongchang], and who left with us for T'eng-Yueh [Tengyue], said that he had passed through the place in July; that at that time there were scarcely any inhabitants left, and that the dead bodies were lying about unburied. Now he said that the disease had ceased at that place, and had moved in a southerly direction to Niu-wa where it was raging. In describing the symptoms, the people said that a lump like a boil, . . . suddenly appeared on almost any part of the body. In twenty-four hours, [the victim] died. (Gill 1883: 272)

Southwestern counties suffered greatly during the Muslim Rebellion and were also hit hard by plague (Table 8). During the war, epidemics appeared up and down the highway between Simao and Kunming, striking Ning'er in 1860 and 1862, Talang in 1861 and 1865, and Yuanjiang in 1867 (*Pu'erfu zhigao* 1900, 3: 8a; *Yuanjiang zhigao* 1922, 6: 1). Louis de Carné, a member of the Laos-to-Kunming expedition led by

TABLE 8
Recorded Epidemics in Southwestern Yunnan, 1860–90

Year	Location	Source consulted
1860	Ning'er	*Pu'erfu zhigao* 1900, 3: 8a
1861	Talang	*Pu'erfu zhigao* 1900, 3: 8a
1862	Ning'er	*Pu'erfu zhigao* 1900, 3: 8b
1865	Talang	*Pu'erfu zhigao* 1900, 3: 8b
1867	Yuanjiang	*Yuanjiang zhigao* 1922, 6: 1
1871	Simao	Rocher 1879: map folder
1871	Ning'er	Rocher 1879: map folder
1871	Talang	Rocher 1879: map folder
1871	Yuanjiang	Rocher 1879: map folder
1871	Xinping	Rocher 1879: map folder
1874	Ning'er	*Pu'erfu zhigao* 1900, 3: 8a
1875	Yuanjiang	*Yunnan tongzhi* 1894, n.p.
1876–77	Jingdong	*Jingdongxian zhigao* 1923, 2: 134
1890	Xinping	*Xinpingxian zhi* 1934, 15: n.p.

TABLE 9
Recorded Epidemics in Eastern-Central Yunnan, 1856–76

Year	Location	Source consulted
1856–74	Chenggong	*Chenggongxian zhi* 1885, 4: 48b
1863	Kunming	*(Xu) Yunnan tongzhigao* 1901, 2: 24a; *Kunmingxian zhi* 1939, 7: 7a
1865	Kunming	*(Xu) Yunnan tongzhigao* 1901, 2: 24a; *Kunmingxian zhi* 1939, 7: 7a
1871–72	Kunming	Rocher 1879: map folder
1871–72	Xi'e	Rocher 1879: map folder
1871–72	Xinxing	Rocher 1879: map folder
1871–72	Kunyang	Rocher 1879: map folder
1871–72	Chenggong	Rocher 1879: map folder
1871–72	Songming	Rocher 1879: map folder
1871–72	Fumin	Rocher 1879: map folder
1872–73	Kunming	Rocher 1879: map folder
1872–73	Songming	Rocher 1879: map folder
1872–73	Yanglin	Rocher 1879: map folder
1872–73	Chenggong	Rocher 1879: map folder
1872–73	Anning	Rocher 1879: map folder
1872–73	Fumin	Rocher 1879: map folder
1872–73	Kunyang	Rocher 1879: map folder
1872–73	Jiangchuan	Rocher 1879: map folder
1872–73	Hexi	Rocher 1879: map folder
1872–73	Tonghai	Rocher 1879: map folder
1872–73	Ningzhou	Rocher 1879: map folder
1872–73	Heyang	*Yunnan tongzhi* 1894, n.p.
1875–76	Kunming	*Kunmingxian zhi* 1939, 7: 7b

Doudart de Lagrée, witnessed this epidemic in the town of Yuanjiang, later noting that "Epidemics are permanently there. . . . I continually saw coffins carried along the streets by four men; perfumed rods, alight, placed around the lid, exhaling a slight smoke as they passed" (Carné 1982 [1872]: 243). The town of Simao, which had once contained an estimated thirty thousand people, was almost deserted when the de Lagrée expedition passed through, and "there does not remain one house in twenty" (ibid.: 219). The Pu'er prefectural capital at Ning'er was even more deserted, with only one street inhabited (ibid.: 227).

Gazetteers indicate that epidemics also occurred in eastern Yunnan during the Muslim Rebellion, although narrative descriptions of their effects are lacking (Table 9). Chenggong county to the east of Kunming experienced periodic epidemics between 1856 and 1874 (*Chenggongxian zhi* 1885, 4: 48b). Kunming city itself had an outbreak in 1863 and again in 1865 ([Xu] *Yunnan tongzhigao* 1901, 2: 24a). During his tour of eastern Yunnan between 1871 and 1873, Emile Rocher noted that plague was widespread in the counties surrounding Dianchi Lake (Rocher 1879, 2: map folder). Plague also appears to have been prevalent in counties of northeastern Yunnan located along highways leading to Guizhou, Sichuan, and Guangxi (Table 10).

Epidemiological investigations made in the 1950's suggest that plague may have occurred in southeastern Yunnan during the Muslim Rebellion and that it was almost certainly present in the area between 1871 and 1873, when Emile Rocher passed through (*SYLXS* 1982: 871–72, 874, 878; Rocher 1879, 2: map folder). (See Table 11.) Hardest hit were the towns of Jianshui, Shiping, and Mengzi. Accounts of these epidemics in gazetteers evoke images of immense suffering. The compiler of the Mengzi gazetteer, for example, describes the following scene:

Following the [1873] epidemic, the two-year-old son of the Su family of Lin'an sat on the road wailing. His cry was terribly tragic. By his side sat his nurse. With tears streaming down her face, she said, "The Su family consisted of twelve people, but nine of them have already died. There used to be a daughter-in-law and myself to care for this son but today the daughter-in-law died and only I am left." ([Xu] *Mengzixian zhi* 1961 [1911], 12: 43b)[25]

After 1871, towns in the southeastern section of the province continued to experience periodic outbreaks of plague for the next twenty to thirty years: Jianshui from 1872 to 1893, Shiping from 1886 to 1896, and Mengzi from 1873 to 1893 (*Shipingxian zhi* 1938, 34: 18b; [Xu]

TABLE 10

Recorded Epidemics in Northeastern Yunnan, 1863–98

Year	Location	Source consulted
1863	Kunming	(*Xu*) *Yunnan tongzhigao* 1901, 2: 24a; *Kunmingxian zhi* 1939, 7: 7a
1863–64	Luquan	*Luquanxian zhi* 1928, 1: 38b
1864	Zhanyi	*Kunmingxian zhi* 1939, 7: 7b
1865	Kunming	(*Xu*) *Yunnan tongzhigao* 1901, 2: 24a; *Kunmingxian zhi* 1939, 7: 7a
1871	Kunming	Rocher 1879: map folder
1871	Zhenxiong	*Zhenxiongzhou zhi* 1887, 5: 63b
1871–72	Yiliang	Rocher 1879: map folder
1871–72	Lu'nan	Rocher 1879: map folder
1871–72	Luxi	Rocher 1879: map folder
1871–72	Malong	Rocher 1879: map folder
1871–72	Luliang	Rocher 1879: map folder
1871–72	Nanning	Rocher 1879: map folder
1871–72	Xuanwei	Rocher 1879: map folder
1871–72	Dongchuan	Rocher 1879: map folder
1871–72	Zhaotong	Rocher 1879: map folder
1872	Luxi	*Yunnan tongzhi* 1894, n.p.
1872–73	Luxi	Rocher 1879: map folder
1872–73	Luoping	Rocher 1879: map folder
1872–73	Lu'nan	Rocher 1879: map folder
1872–73	Mile	Rocher 1879: map folder
1872–73	Malong	Rocher 1879: map folder
1872–73	Zhanyi	Rocher 1879: map folder
1875–76	Kunming	*Kunmingxian zhi* 1939, 7: 7b
1875–76	Zhaotong	*Zhaotong zhigao* 1924, 12: 16b
1882	Zhanyi	*Zhanyizhou zhi* 1885, 4: 83
1882–92	Luoping	*Luopingxian zhi* 1933, 1: 76
1892–93	Zhaotong	*Yunnan tongzhi* 1894, n.p.
1892–93	Dongchuan	*Yunnan tongzhi* 1894, n.p.
1894	Zhanyi	*Kunmingxian zhi* 1939, 7: 7b
1897–98	Luliang	*Luliangxian zhigao* 1915, 1: 7a–7b

Mengzixian zhi 1961 [1911], 12: 43b; *Yunnan tongzhi* 1894: n.p.). Plague appears to have killed large numbers of people in the southeastern subregion during these years: a tenth of the population of Jianshui was reported to have died of *yangzibing* in the 1870's ([*Xuxiu*] *Jianshui-xian zhigao* 1920, 10: 22a). Deaths due to plague in Mengzi between 1873 and 1893 were said to exceed ten thousand ([*Xu*] *Mengzixian zhi* 1961 [1911], 12: 43b). As one foreign observer noted, "Death travels fast in Mengtsz [Mengzi]. Thousands of victims yearly made by plague require to be buried" (Inspectorate General, *Customs Medical Reports* 1894, No. 48: 36).

TABLE 11
Recorded Epidemics in Southeastern Yunnan, 1871–93

Year	Location	Source consulted
1871	Shiping	Rocher 1879: map folder
1871	Jianshui	Rocher 1879: map folder
1872–73	Jianshui	Rocher 1879: map folder
1872–73	Mengzi	Rocher 1879: map folder
1872–73	Wenshan	Rocher 1879: map folder
1872–73	Ami	Rocher 1879: map folder
1872–73	Qiubei	Rocher 1879: map folder
1872–93	Jianshui	*Yunnan tongzhi* 1894: n.p.
1873	Wenshan	*Yunnan tongzhi* 1894: n.p.
1873	Mengzi	(*Xu*) *Mengzixian zhi* 1961 [1911], 12: 43b
1873–93	Mengzi	(*Xu*) *Mengzixian zhi* 1961 [1911], 12: 43b
1874–75	Qiubei	*Qiubeixian zhi* 1926: n.p.
1875	Mengzi	Rocher 1879: map folder
1876–78	Qiubei	*Qiubeixian zhi* 1926: n.p.

Conclusion

Plague may have been present in western Yunnan long before the late eighteenth century, but it did not reach epidemic proportions until demographic and economic changes in the province created an environment that allowed for its extensive spread through the human population. Such conditions emerged during the upswing in Yungui's regional economy between 1750 and 1800. In the newly emergent boomtowns of late-eighteenth-century Yunnan, conditions were ideal for an explosion in the plague-carrying yellow-chested rat population. Moreover, economic expansion and the growth of cities in the region stimulated long-distance trade. As the number of traders traveling between western and eastern Yunnan increased, so did the possibility that the plague bacillus and its hosts would be carried from enzootic centers in Lijiang prefecture to areas previously unaffected. This may well have happened between 1772 and 1830, years when unusually large numbers of epidemics are recorded in Yunnan's local gazetteers.

Although we can never be certain that bubonic plague was responsible for these epidemics, Shi Daonan's poem and Gu Chun's memorial strongly suggest that it was. Moreover, the geographical pattern of epidemics seems to indicate spread of disease at the end of the eigh-

teenth century from the regional periphery in western Yunnan to its
core in the eastern part of the province. The initial outbreak in Heqing
was in 1772, yet Dali was not affected until 1796. Kunming had its first
epidemic in 1803, and the disease did not spread to Jianshui until 1810.
This slow progression from one jurisdiction to another underscores the
difficulties imposed on transport by Yunnan's topography; it also high-
lights the extent to which the regional system of Yungui was still devel-
oping. By 1850 the province was integrated to such an extent that after
plague broke out it spread rather quickly from Kunming, Dali, and
Mengzi to towns along the major trade routes. Outbreaks of the disease intensified during the years of the Muslim Rebellion. Larger numbers of people moved through Yunnan than ever before, as refugees
and soldiers joined traders and travelers on the highways. The chaotic
conditions in besieged cities and the intensified movement around the
province allowed plague to spread more quickly to a much wider area.

Plague did not spread far beyond the borders of Yunnan in the early
nineteenth century because the Yungui macroregion was not yet well
integrated into an interregional trading system. Although some long-
distance trade did exist in the eighteenth and early nineteenth centuries, a critical level of human movement between Yungui and other
regions had not yet been reached. Over the course of the nineteenth
century, Yunnan was increasingly incorporated into the broader Chinese polity and economy. The intensification of interregional activity
thus engendered allowed plague to spill over the borders of the Yungui macroregion into other areas of southern China, particularly the
Lingnan region to the east.

CHAPTER 2

The Interregional Spread of Plague, 1860-1894

IN THE SECOND half of the nineteenth century, bubonic plague began to appear in Guangxi and Guangdong, the two provinces that make up the Lingnan macroregion.[1] In the 1860's, plague epidemics broke out in towns situated near the Leizhou Peninsula of western Guangdong. Then, in the 1870's and 1880's, the disease was carried to Hainan Island and to towns lying along the southern Guangdong coast. Finally, in the 1890's, plague reached the Pearl River Delta. By the spring of 1894, bubonic plague had reached the major metropolises of Hong Kong and Canton, and from there began spreading to other cities around the world.

When plague first appeared in Hong Kong and Canton, a number of foreign observers were aware of Emile Rocher's account of Yunnan's epidemics during the Muslim Rebellion, and they concluded that the southeastern epidemics had originated in the southwest (Rocher 1879, 1: 75; 2: 279–81). In a report on the 1894 plague in Canton, for example, Dr. Alexander Rennie speculated that merchants had carried the disease overland from Yunnan to Guangdong through Guangxi or the border areas of Tonkin[2] (Inspectorate General, *Customs Medical Reports* 1894, No. 48: 65–67). William Simpson (1905: 56), an epidemiologist who studied plague in Hong Kong after the 1894 outbreak there, also made a connection between the Yunnan epidemics and the appearance of plague in Guangdong. Simpson disagreed with Rennie over the mechanism that had brought the disease from the southwest to the coast, pointing out that the distance between Yunnan and Guangdong was so great and the amount of trade so insignificant that the disease was unlikely to have been diffused by commerce. Because Rocher had reported plague being present at the height of the Muslim Rebellion, Simpson speculated that it was less likely to have been imported into Guangdong by traders than by troops returning to the area after fighting in Yunnan.

The thesis that troop movements rather than trade was the reason for the spread of the disease from Yunnan to Lingnan has been accepted at face value in subsequent descriptions of the origins of the third pandemic. R. Pollitzer (1954: 152), a League of Nations epidemiologist who conducted research on plague in China in the 1930's, simply restated Simpson's speculation. William McNeill, in his classic *Plagues and Peoples*, embellishes the story, maintaining that "Chinese troops were sent across the Salween [in the far western periphery of Yunnan] to suppress the [Muslim] rebels, and being unfamiliar with the risks of bubonic infection, contracted the disease and carried it back with them across the river into the rest of China" (1976: 135). McNeill overlooks the incredible distance between the Leizhou Peninsula and the Salween (Nu) River (in western Yunnan), and thus the implausibility of direct communication between the two.

Although earlier researchers have made a connection between the Yunnan epidemics and the appearance of plague in the Lingnan region, the historical reasons for its spread have not been thoroughly examined. When the path of the disease is systematically tracked and embedded in the local history of the areas it passed through, it becomes clear that in the mid-nineteenth century there was a heightened level of movement through the border areas between Yunnan, Guangxi, Tonkin, and the Leizhou Peninsula.[3] This intensification of travel was due to commercial, military, and bandit activity, any one of which was sufficient cause for the spread of plague across macroregional boundaries. Plague may have been carried to western Guangdong from southeastern Yunnan by militiamen returning home or by migrants fleeing the violence of the Muslim Rebellion, as William Simpson believed. It is also possible, as Alexander Rennie contended, that traders spread the disease because commerce, particularly the trade in domestic opium, continued even during the worst years of disorder and rebellion. As in the southwest, the critical factor allowing for the spread of plague was not the identity of the actual agents (merchants, soldiers, bandits, or refugees) who effected its transmission but significant changes in patterns of transport and travel over the course of the mid-nineteenth century.

The Development of the Yunnan-Lingnan Opium Trade

At the beginning of the eighteenth century, Yunnan was still relatively isolated from the coastal provinces to the east. With some exceptions (Dali marble, Pu'er tea, minerals and precious stones), no commodity could bear the cost of overland transport over the large distances and difficult terrain that separated Yunnan from the rest of the empire. The long-distance trade that did exist was oriented predominantly toward Guiyang in central Guizhou and Chongqing in Sichuan rather than the West River system that leads into Guangxi and Guangdong (Map 13).[4] After the Qing government constructed a road from Chenggong in Yunnan to Tianyang in Guangxi in 1729, the travel time between Kunming and Nanning was cut in half. As a consequence, the West River route quickly became the primary route to Yunnan from Guangxi and Guangdong (J. Lee 1993: 97, 101). Moreover, evidence suggests that, in the middle of the nineteenth century, travel between Yunnan and the Lingnan region along the West River and its tributaries intensified yet again. The single most important reason for this increase in trade was the development of a Cantonese distribution network in Guangxi and Guangdong for opium grown in Yunnan.

Long valued as a medicinal herb, opium had been cultivated in western China at least since the Tang dynasty (Spence 1975: 151). Prior to the nineteenth century, it was grown on a limited basis in the mountains of Yunnan (Lin Manhong 1985: 183–87). The spread of opium addiction among the general Chinese population following the introduction of Malwa and Patna opium into China by English traders created a large domestic market for the drug. The foreign drug was costly, however, and was out of reach for most Chinese.[5] Opium grown in Yunnan was considered to be superior to that of other provinces. The cheaper price relative to the foreign drug and higher quality relative to other domestically grown opium created a great demand for the Yunnan product throughout southern China.

It is impossible to know exactly when opium began to be planted in Yunnan on a large scale or when the Yunnan-Lingnan trade in opium solidified.[6] The first record of opium cultivation in Yunnan dates to 1736, but production for the domestic market appears to have devel-

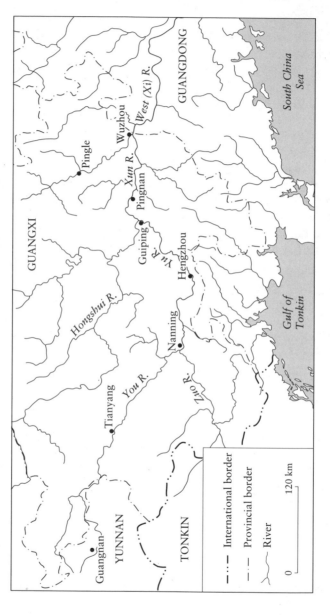

MAP 13. The West River system.

oped only in the 1820's (Lin Manhong 1985: 183–87). In 1836, Xu Naiji mentioned that opium was being grown in several southern provinces, including Yunnan (Spence 1975: 151). By the mid-1830's, opium production in Yunnan was reported to be "several thousand chests annually" (Grandstaff 1979: 73). In 1847, the yield of domestically grown opium in Guangdong was estimated to be between 8,000 and 10,000 piculs (370,000–604,500 kg), and, as Spence (1975: 152) points out, it must have been much higher in western China, where growing conditions were superior. Archibald Colquhoun (1883, 1: 192) was told in 1882 that the Yunnan-Lingnan trade in opium had existed for "two generations." Sometime in the mid-nineteenth century, then, Yunnan opium began to be widely traded in Guangxi and Guangdong.

Opium traders used several routes to transport the drug between Yunnan and Lingnan (Map 14). They carried it overland, from either Kunming or Mengzi, along various roads in the eastern part of Yunnan to Bose in Guangxi (Kunming–Guangnan–Bose direct, or Mengzi-Wenshan–Guangnan–Bose; see Royal Asiatic Society 1893–94: 69–73). Yet another heavily traveled route went from Kunming to Bose via Luoping.[7] According to surveyors affiliated with the nineteenth-century Royal Asiatic Society, the Luoping route was used exclusively for the transport of opium for export to Guangxi and Guangdong; all other traffic took alternate routes (ibid.). From Bose, a small amount was distributed throughout southwestern Guangxi; the rest was transported to Nanning, where it was then either carried overland to Qinzhou and Beihai (Pakhoi) or shipped farther downriver to Wuzhou and the West River, and eventually to the intricate water transport network of the Pearl River Delta.[8]

A second route from Yunnan to Lingnan followed the Red River farther south, through Tonkin to Haiphong. In the nineteenth century, the upper reaches of the Red River were not navigable, and opium bought at Mengzi had to be carried by mule train to the market town of Manhao, 40 miles south of Mengzi. From there, shallow-bottomed boats departed for the Vietnamese border town of Laojie (Laokai). The cargo was transferred to larger boats and moved down the river to Haiphong, where it was transshipped to Beihai. Finally, coastal junks carried the drug to Canton (Inspectorate General, *Decennial Reports* 1882–91: 665–80).[9]

Most of the opium grown in eastern Yunnan was shipped via Bose down the You and West Rivers; that grown in western Yunnan moved down the Red River and was then carried by junks across the Tonkin

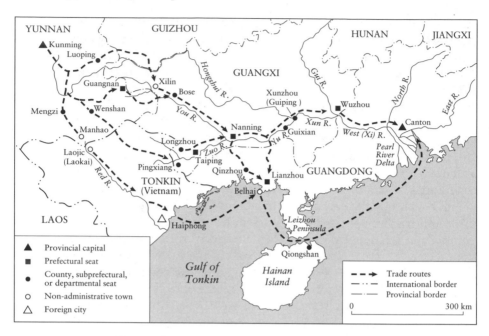

MAP 14. Yunnan-Lingnan trade routes, ca. 1840.

Gulf. An overland route also existed along the border region between Yunnan, Tonkin, and Guangxi (Tōa Dōbunkai 1919, 2: 451–63). In the nineteenth century this was a peripheral, mountainous area inhabited largely by hill tribes, and for this reason it was favored by opium smugglers. Caravan traders moved from Mengzi through southeastern Yunnan or through the upper Red River valley into northern Tonkin along a network of paths that led eventually to Pingxiang on the Guangxi border. (Pingxiang was also the port of entry for Vietnamese tributary missions to Beijing.) The caravans then made their way to Longzhou and Taiping, and from there either went downriver to Nanning or overland to Qinzhou, Beihai, and Lianzhou (Inspectorate General, *Decennial Reports* 1882–91: 661).[10]

All the routes between Canton and Yunnan were long, and travel along them was exceedingly difficult (see Map 14). The journey from the Xilin terminus of the You River to Canton was some 830 miles along a waterway filled with rocks, sandbars, and rapids (Inspectorate General, *Decennial Reports* 1882–91: 647). The trip from Canton to Nanning alone, along the most navigable part of the river, took about 30 days (ibid.: 654); from Canton to Bose took about 45 days by large boat (Royal Asiatic Society 1893–94: map, p. 69) and about 75 days by smaller craft (Inspectorate General, *Decennial Reports* 1882–91: 665). Transporting goods overland from Bose to Mengzi took approximately 18 days, and from Bose to Kunming, about 22 days. Shipping goods downriver from Bose to Canton took only 18 days, but torrential currents during the summer rainy season made many parts of the river impassable (Royal Asiatic Society 1893–94: 69). Travelers were understandably reluctant to travel along sections of the river during the malaria season (ibid.: 73).

Merchants involved in the lucrative opium trade were among the few souls willing to undertake the long and dangerous journey into the interior and back. The unit price of opium was so high that it easily covered the high transportation costs (Lin Manhong 1985: 436–38). Archibald Colquhoun, who traveled along the West River system through Guangxi to Yunnan in 1882, noted that the opium trade was "in the hands of a small number of adventurous trading spirits, who face the dangers and fatigues of the journey [from Canton to Yunnan] undauntedly for the sake of the heavy profit made" (1883, 1: 148). These traders established outposts along the West River and its tributaries, building *huiguan* (native place associations) and setting up pawnshops to facilitate credit transactions (*Boseting zhi* 1891, 5: 10; Colquhoun 1883, 1: 126, 220, 266, 316). By the late nineteenth century, Cantonese merchants were by far the most numerous in Yunnan, and Cantonese native-place associations were located in five of the six most important commercial centers of the province (Metzgar 1973: 24). The Yunnan-Lingnan trade was almost totally controlled by the Cantonese, and they were the group most likely to use the West River route (Royal Asiatic Society 1893–94: 61).

Given the fragmentary evidence available, it is difficult to determine when Yunnan opium began to be transported to Guangxi and Guangdong. It is equally difficult to measure the degree to which opium stimulated movement between the two regions. The evidence suggests, however, that consolidation of the Yunnan-Lingnan opium trade dates to about 1840. As a consequence, in the decade that followed there was an intensification of traffic along the roads and waterways that linked Yunnan with the coast, particularly the West River and its tributaries.

Mid-Nineteenth-Century Disruptions Along the West River and the Rise of Beihai

Throughout the 1840's, the West River route via Bose and Nanning remained the primary conduit between Canton and Yunnan. As China plunged into the disorder and dissension of the 1850's and 1860's, traffic along sections of the Xun River in Guangxi and the West River in Guangdong was increasingly disrupted, first by banditry and secret-society activity and then by rebellion and revolt. Cantonese merchants seeking alternative routes into Yunnan increasingly came to use those that passed through the town of Beihai, situated near the Leizhou Peninsula (see Map 14).

Nineteenth-century Guangxi was a notorious haven for both seafaring and riverine pirates and also for triad society members.[11] Early in the century, piracy had been largely limited to coastal areas, particularly the Qinzhou region of western Guangdong (Murray 1987: 6–20). With the expansion of the opium trade (both domestic and foreign), piracy in the interior increased (Laai 1950: 62–73). To protect themselves against robbery and kidnapping, itinerant merchants formed networks of triad cells along the West River system. Such societies engendered their own forms of criminal activity, operating smuggling, petty banditry, and protection rackets. During the first half of the nineteenth century, merchants could buy protection from both the bandits and the secret societies and still continue to use the waterways. Travel along the Yu, Xun, and West Rivers was dangerous and difficult but not impossible if one had connections with the underworld.

The Taiping rebels were another matter. The Taiping Heavenly Kingdom (*Taiping tianguo*) had its origins in Guixian and Guiping, two counties lying along the Xun River (see Map 14). Before the rebels began their march northward, away from Guangxi and toward the rich provinces of the lower Yangzi River valley, their clashes with Qing imperial troops effectively disrupted the flow of goods and people along the Xun and West Rivers (Jen 1973: 71–79; Laai, Michael, and Sherman 1962: map 1; Zhang Haipeng 1983: map 18). Between November 1850 and January 1851, the Taipings controlled the part of the Xun River that flowed through Guiping county, although Qing troops had managed to blockade sections farther east (Zhang Haipeng 1983: map 19). In February 1851, largely as a result of their inability to control communications along the entire Xun River, the rebels were forced to give up their riverine base in Guiping county. After numerous skirmishes with imperial troops, in 1852 they began their expedition northward.

The departure of the Taipings from Guangxi did not mean that traffic along the Xun and West Rivers returned to normal. In the summer of 1850, at the same time the Taiping rebels began congregating in the districts of Guixian and Guiping, triad organizations along other parts of the West River were beginning to revolt (Wakeman 1972: 38). Triad mobilization against the Qing reached its peak in the summer of 1854, when tens of thousands of "Red Turbans" captured towns in the Pearl River Delta and threatened to take the regional metropolis of Canton. The Qing managed to recover most of the territory in the delta by the winter of 1854, and imperial troops forced the remaining rebels to retreat back along the West River. By June 1855 the insurgents had fled as far as Guiping, where they remained headquartered for the next three years. Between 1855 and 1858 the rebels expanded the territory they controlled along the Xun River, eventually taking Hengzhou, Pingle, Nanning, and Wuzhou (see Map 13). The Qing were not able to reclaim the districts lying along the Xun River until 1860, and normal transport conditions did not resume until 1861.

During the last few years of the 1840's and throughout the 1850's, revolt and rebellion effectively blocked off large segments of the main avenue between Yunnan and the provinces of Guangxi and Guangdong. Hostilities along the West River and its tributaries forced traders to use other routes into the southwest. There were three other ways to get to Yunnan from Canton: along the You River via the western Guangdong coast and Nanning; along the Red River via Haiphong; and overland from western Guangdong through Tonkin along the Sino-Vietnamese border (see Map 14). These alternate routes all converged on a newly thriving entrepôt, the town of Beihai in western Guangdong.

The town of Beihai emerged in the second half of the nineteenth century as a major center for the Yunnan-Lingnan opium trade. Located on a small peninsula that jutted southward from the Lianzhou prefectural seat, and just west of the larger Leizhou Peninsula, the town was ideally situated to serve as a transit post for maritime, riverine, and overland transport (Map 15). A natural harbor, surrounded by land on the south and the east, provided easy access even for large vessels, and sandbars on the north and west provided safe anchorage during severe storms (Inspectorate General, *Decennial Reports* 1882–91: 644). Beihai was a convenient port of call for junks crossing the Gulf

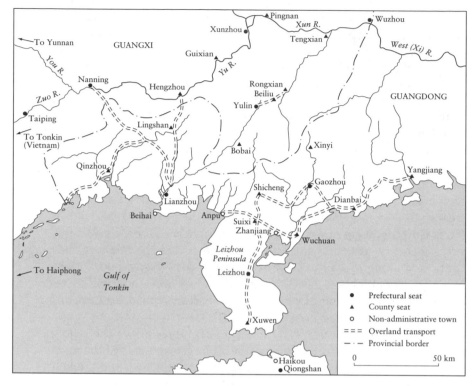

MAP 15. Transport routes in western Guangdong, ca. 1850.

of Tonkin from Haiphong. A road ran north to Lianzhou; from there goods could be shipped by river to Yulin and then carried overland to Beiliu and Rongxian (Colquhoun 1883, 1: 73). Similarly, goods transported from Beihai to Qinzhou could be carried overland to Nanning and then up the You River to Yunnan (Royal Asiatic Society 1893–94: 105). To the east of Beihai is a level plain over which wheelbarrows and bullock carts conveyed goods to villages on the Leizhou Peninsula (Inspectorate General, *Decennial Reports* 1882–91: 649). Beyond Anpu, which could be reached both overland and by boat from Beihai, a hilly road led to counties situated in Leizhou prefecture (Tōa Dōbunkai 1919, 1: 591–618). Itinerant traders from Beihai also carried goods along the overland paths that extended from western Guangdong into northern Tonkin.[12]

Despite its obvious transport advantages, Beihai appears not to have been a major center of trade before the mid-nineteenth century. The town was reportedly established in 1852 by some merchants from Canton who set up a wholesaling depot there (Simpson 1905: 56).[13] If Beihai does indeed date to the early 1850's, its establishment may be related to the disruptions to trade along the Xun and West Rivers during this same decade. I cannot prove that such a linkage exists, but the timing and purpose of Beihai's supposed origins are intriguing. Faced with great unrest along the West River, Cantonese merchants involved in the domestic opium trade may have sought new routes between Yunnan and Lingnan so as to avoid the most violent sections of the river. For a time in the 1850's, the alternate routes into Yunnan, while plagued by chronic banditry, were free of the military blockades and active warfare found along the inland waterways to the east.[14] If trade between Yunnan and Canton continued during the tumultuous 1850's, it seems most likely that opium merchants would have elected to travel along the byways in western Lingnan that avoided the West and Xun Rivers altogether.

There is some evidence that the domestic opium trade did thrive during the Taiping and triad disturbances in Guangxi and the Muslim Rebellion in Yunnan.[15] Disorder may even have allowed the Yunnan-Lingnan opium trade to increase because, with the breakdown of Qing authority, the illicit drug could be more openly grown and traded. A truce negotiated in 1862 between Dali and Kunming included a provision allowing for safe passage of caravan traders through the province. Chinese traders told Thomas Cooper, an Englishman traveling through western Yunnan in 1868, that according to orders given by the Muslim leader Du Wenxiu, the Muslim army would only plunder an area for three days in a row, so traders waited until the fourth day to travel. In his memoirs, Cooper wrote:

Thus during intervals of warfare, considerable trade is carried on between Moslem and Imperial Yunnan in skins, *opium*, iron pots, cotton goods, and tobacco, on which both governments levy duties, the Mahomedan king fostering trade as much as possible, both by the imposition of light duties and a rigorous administration of justice, to which the traders bore ample testimony. Indeed, a flourishing trade had existed for two years prior to my arrival [i.e., since 1866], Imperial Chinese having had free access to Mahomedan territory and vice versa. (1871b: 330; emphasis added)

John Anderson (1972 [1876]: 42), who accompanied the Sladen expedition to Tengyue in 1868, found that opium from Yunnan was still available in Burmese markets in 1868, although Cooper (1869: 150–51) had noted that other Chinese goods could not be found there. He also observed that the Muslim Rebellion had cut off the supply of Yunnan opium to Sichuan but that the trade was revived between 1864 and 1865 (ibid.). It seems likely that opium merchants from Guangdong continued to trade in Yunnan as well. This hypothesis is given credence by Archibald Colquhoun's (1883, 1: 130) comment that during the 1850's the "fugitive" trade between Yunnan and Canton continued, by which he presumably meant the trade in opium.

Expansion of the domestic opium trade from Yunnan to Lingnan, combined with the complexity and scope of disorder along the West River between 1850 and 1860, meant that there was an unusually high degree of movement between western Guangdong and southeastern Yunnan during this decade. The trade routes that passed from Mengzi and Kunming in Yunnan to Beihai near the Leizhou Peninsula were heavily traveled not only by opium traders but also by bandits and Qing government troops (see Map 14). Before the Qing restored order in Guangxi in the 1860's, outlaw gangs moved about relatively freely on the Chinese side of the border (Laffey 1972; 1975; and 1976). Even after the Qing successfully forced the bandits into Tonkin, they occasionally ventured back into western Guangdong or Guangxi before being chased back into Vietnamese territory by imperial troops stationed along the frontier (Laffey 1975: 45–49). This intensified movement by bandits, soldiers, and, above all, opium smugglers provided the necessary precondition for the spread of plague from Yunnan to the Lingnan region.

The Diffusion of Plague from Yunnan to Lingnan

The chronology of plague epidemics along the Yunnan-Lingnan trade routes suggests that the disease was first carried overland from Wenshan county (in Kaihua prefecture) in southeastern Yunnan to the Guangxi-Tonkin border town of Longzhou (Table 12 and Map 16). In the 1950's, epidemiological researchers determined that plague had been present in the area around Wenshan in the early 1860's. Wenshan apparently experienced an epidemic in 1861–62, Maguan in 1865–66, and Malipo in 1866 (SYLXS 1982: 871, 872, 874, and 878). Plague reached Longzhou in 1866, probably carried overland through the Yunnan–Tonkin–Guangxi border region (ibid.: 1684). Historical records for the border areas of Tonkin are scarce, and there are no specific reports of plague in this region (Ortholan 1908: 633–38). Ac-

TABLE 12
Recorded Epidemics Along Yunnan-Lingnan Trade Routes, 1861–67

Year	Location	Source consulted
1861–62	Wenshan	SYLXS 1982: 872
1864	Longan	Longanxian zhi 1934, 1: 4a
1865	Wuyuan	Wuyuanxian zhi 1914, 10: 34a
1865	Qianjiang	Qianjiangxian zhi 1935, 5: 202
1865–66	Maguan	SYLXS 1982: 874
1866	Malipo	SYLXS 1982: 878
1866	Longzhou	SYLXS 1982: 1684
1867	Shanglin	Shanglinxian zhi 1899 [1876], 1: 109
1867	Beihai	Inspectorate General, Customs Medical Reports 1882, No. 24: 31

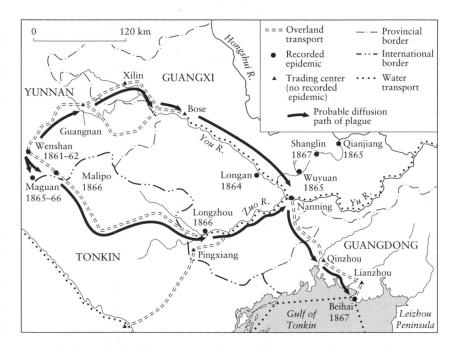

MAP 16. Recorded epidemics along Yunnan-Lingnan trade routes, 1861–67.

cording to Ella Laffey (1975: 51), the area suffered severe depopulation in the 1860's and 1870's. This loss of population was so great that in the 1880's the French, Chinese, and Vietnamese armies could not find any coolies to carry their supplies. Laffey assumes that high mortality resulted from fighting among the many bandit gangs that roamed the area in the 1860's and 1870's. No doubt many villagers in the region suffered at the hands of outlaws, but there is also the possibility that plague was moving through the region from southeastern Yunnan to western Guangdong. Alexander Rennie's hypothesis that the disease spread to the Leizhou Peninsula from Yunnan via northern Tonkin is given credence by Chinese sources, which state that the disease came to Guangxi from Tonkin during the Tongzhi reign (1862–74; see *Shundexian zhi* 1929, 23: 16; *Yangjiangxian zhi* 1925, 37: 43).

Plague may also have been moving down the You River during this period (see Map 16). Plague epidemics began to be recorded for towns along the You River and its tributaries in the 1860's. Plague is reported to have begun in Shanglin county, located about 55 km north of Nanning, in 1867, and to have continued for the next thirteen years (*Shanglinxian zhi* 1899 [1876], 1: 10a). In addition to this epidemic, which is identified as *shuyi* (plague), numerous other gazetteers record *yi* (epidemics) around the same time. Longan county, located on the You River, had an epidemic outbreak in 1864 (*Longanxian zhi* 1934, 1: 4a). Wuyuan, located about halfway between Nanning and Shanglin on a tributary of the You River, experienced an epidemic in 1865 (*Wuyuanxian zhi* 1914, 10: 34a). Qianjiang, on the Hongshui River northeast of Shanglin, also had an unidentified outbreak of epidemic disease in 1865 (*Qianjiangxian zhi* 1935, 5: 202). The proximity of these counties to a place where *shuyi* is said to have been present suggests that the *yi* recorded in the gazetteers were actually outbreaks of plague.

In 1867, the same year that plague appeared in Shanglin county, the disease emerged in Beihai (Inspectorate General, *Customs Medical Reports* 1882, No. 24: 31; *SYLXS* 1982: 1487). Plague may have spread to Beihai via Nanning and Qinzhou. In the 1880's, foreign doctors resident in Beihai noted that outbreaks of plague there usually followed the appearance of the disease in Bose, Longzhou, and Nanning (Inspectorate General, *Customs Medical Reports* 1889–90, No. 39: 15; 1890–91, No. 41: 32). Nanning had its first recorded epidemic in 1889, but a resident French priest reported that plague had been present there for many years before (ibid. 1889–90, No. 39: 15).

During the last three decades of the nineteenth century, plague con-

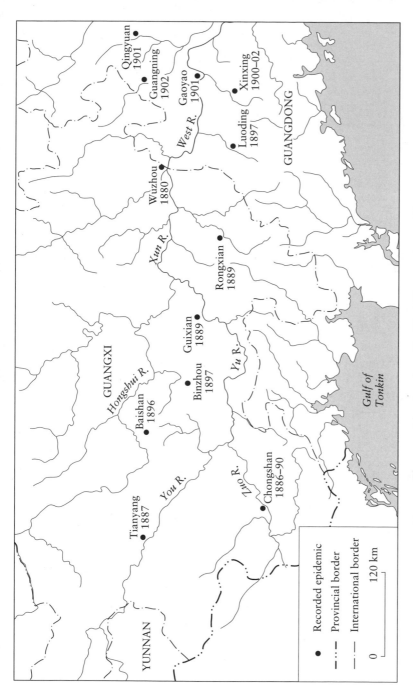

MAP 17. Plague epidemics along the West River system, 1880–1902.

TABLE 13

Recorded Epidemics Along the West River System, 1880–1902

Year	Location	Source consulted
1880	Wuzhou	*SYLXS* 1982: 1684
1886–90	Chongshan	*Chongshanxian zhi* 1937, 5: n.p.
1887	Tianyang	*SYLXS* 1982: 1684
1889	Guixian	*SYLXS* 1982: 1684
1889	Rongxian	*Rongxian zhi* 1897, 2: 11b
1896	Baishan	*SYLXS* 1982: 1684
1897	Binzhou	*Binyangxian zhi* 1948, 6: 578
1897	Luoding	*SYLXS* 1982: 1582
1900–1902	Xinxing	*SYLXS* 1982: 1585
1901	Gaoyao	*(Xuantong) Gaoyaoxian zhi* 1938, 13: 45
1901	Qingyuan	*SYLXS* 1982: 1587
1902	Guangning	*SYLXS* 1982: 1590

NOTE: Only first recorded epidemics are listed. See *SYLXS* (1982: 1684–88) for lists of reported plague epidemics in subsequent years.

tinued to spread from Yunnan to Beihai and along the Yu and Xun Rivers in Guangxi province (Table 13). The disease was particularly widespread in Guangxi in the 1880's and 1890's (Map 17). Although plague was recorded periodically in other districts of Guangxi as well, it never took hold in Guangxi to the extent that it did in Yunnan. This is probably because the environmental conditions in much of Guangxi do not provide a favorable habitat for the primary plague-carrying rodent of southern China, the yellow-chested rat (*Rattus flavipectus*). Plague continued to appear sporadically in western Guangxi until 1944, but most outbreaks were a result of the disease being imported from elsewhere.

The Diffusion of Plague from Beihai to Central and Eastern Guangdong

In contrast to the interior of Guangxi, conditions in western Guangdong were ideal for sustaining both the yellow-chested rat and the Asiatic rat flea (*Xenopsylla cheopis*). A 1950's study of rodents in the area around Beihai and on the Leizhou Peninsula showed that the yellow-chested rat constituted 95 percent of all commensal rodents in the area (*SYLXS* 1982: 1469). Indeed, contemporary epidemiologists have identified this area as one of China's natural plague reservoirs

(Ji Shuli 1988: 66). These favorable environmental conditions may account for the repeated epidemics Beihai suffered after 1867. Beihai had annual outbreaks of plague between 1871 and 1877. The disease broke out again in 1882 and then continued to appear in Beihai with some frequency in the twentieth century (*SYLXS* 1982: 1487).

In the 1870's and 1880's, Cantonese merchants traveling to and from Yunnan continued to use the alternate routes that passed through Beihai even after the Qing government had suppressed the myriad revolts along the West River. This preference was linked to the workings of the internal-transit tax system (*lijin*) and to the establishment of steamship service between Beihai and Hong Kong. Provincial and local authorities introduced *lijin* taxes into Guangdong province in the summer of 1858, and into Guangxi in the fall of that same year (Beal 1958: 43). In the early stages of the system, the collection depots were located along the sections of the Xun and West Rivers between Nanning, Wuzhou, and Canton (see Map 14); in the 1860's there were seven stations between Wuzhou and Canton alone (Mann 1987: 118, 125).[16] Before 1891, however, there were very few *lijin* posts west of Nanning, and as a result transportation between Yunnan and Nanning was relatively cheap (Inspectorate General, *Decennial Reports* 1882–91: 655). To avoid paying transit fees downriver, merchants preferred to transport their cargo overland from Nanning to the coastal town of Qinzhou and then on to Beihai (ibid.: 547, 661).

Although Beihai had previously been linked to major seaports along the South China coast by the indigenous junk trade, its relationship to towns of the Pearl River Delta was transformed after its designation as a treaty port in 1876 and the establishment of steamship service after 1879. Until 1885 steamships only made irregular trips between Beihai and Canton. After 1885 steamer service gradually increased, and by 1891 foreign-operated steamships were running regularly between the two ports (Inspectorate General, *Decennial Reports* 1882–91: 637–40). Whereas it had previously taken a month to travel from Canton to Nanning via the West River, it now took only sixteen days to ship goods to Beihai and then carry them overland to Nanning (ibid.: 654).

The speed afforded by steamers and Beihai's new status as a treaty port, combined with the absence of transit-fee collection stations in western Guangdong and Guangxi, meant that Beihai's importance as a trade entrepôt increased during the last three decades of the nineteenth century. For a number of years, particularly between the 1870's and the 1890's, a considerable portion of the Yunnan-Lingnan trade

TABLE 14

Recorded Epidemics in Western Guangdong and Eastern Guangxi, 1867–1904

Year	Location	Source consulted
1867	Beihai	*SYLXS* 1982: 1487
1871	Qinzhou	*SYLXS* 1982: 1483
1871	Yulin	*Yulinzhou zhi* 1894, 4: 9
1871	Beiliu	*Beiliuxian zhi* 1880, 1: 13a
1872	Suixi	*SYLXS* 1982: 1504
1877	Shicheng	*Shichengxian zhi* 1931, 10: 34b
1879	Zhanjiang	*SYLXS* 1982: 1570
1880	Wuzhou	*SYLXS* 1982: 1880
1880	Lianzhou	*SYLXS* 1982: 1484
1882	Leizhou	*SYLXS* 1982: 1557
1882	Danxian	Lin Shiquan 1989: 100–101
1888	Haikou	*SYLXS* 1982: 1658
1888	Qiongshan	*SYLXS* 1982: 1660
1888	Luchuan	*SYLXS* 1982: 1684
1889	Nanning	Inspectorate General, *Customs Medical Reports* 1889–90, No. 39: 15
1889	Rongxian	*Rongxian zhi* 1897, 2: 11b
1890	Gaozhou	Zheng Xiaoyan 1936 [1901]: preface
1890	Yangjiang	*SYLXS* 1982: 1568
1890	Wuchuan	*Wuchuanxian zhi* 1892 [1888], 10: 50b
1891	Huazhou	*SYLXS* 1982: 1568
1891	Dianbai	*SYLXS* 1982: 1581
1894	Dingan	*SYLXS* 1982: 1661
1900	Lin'gao	*SYLXS* 1982: 1655
1904	Chengmai	*SYLXS* 1982: 1656

NOTE: Only first recorded epidemics are listed. See *SYLXS* (1982: 1455–1680; 1684–88) for lists of reported plague epidemics in subsequent years.

along the You and West Rivers continued to be diverted through the port. Indeed, Beihai became so central to trade with Yunnan that a customs commissioner complained that Canton had to compete with Beihai throughout the 1880's for the eastern Yunnan trade (Inspectorate General, *Decennial Reports*, 1882–91: 547).

Beihai's economic centrality and its location near a natural plague reservoir assured that it would continue to serve as the point of origin for rediffusion of the disease to communities on the Leizhou Peninsula, Hainan Island, the area around Gaozhou prefecture, and the rivers that led into eastern Guangxi (Map 18). From Beihai, plague spread inland to Yulin and Beiliu counties, both of which had epidemics (*yi*) in 1871 (*Beiliuxian zhi* 1880, 1: 13a; *Yulinzhou zhi* 1894, 4: 9). (See Table 14 and Map 18.) In the early 1870's, travelers carried plague along the road leading from Beihai to the Leizhou Peninsula. Suixi county had an outbreak in 1872 (*SYLXS* 1982: 1504). From Suixi the disease fanned out

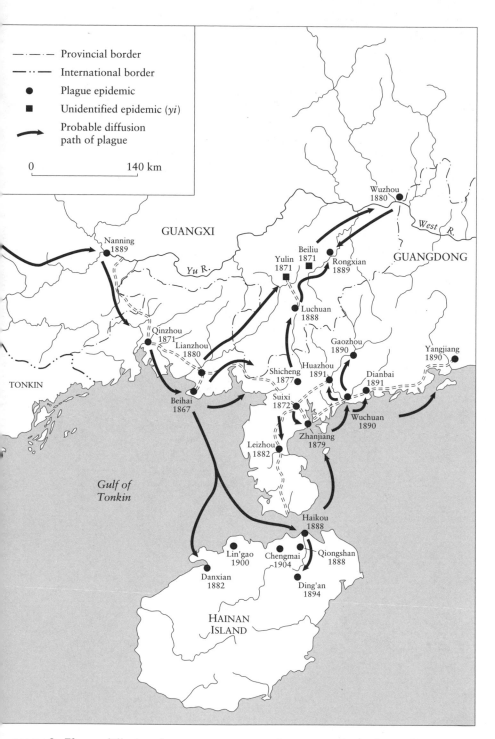

MAP 18. Plague diffusion along transport routes in western Guangdong, 1867–1900.

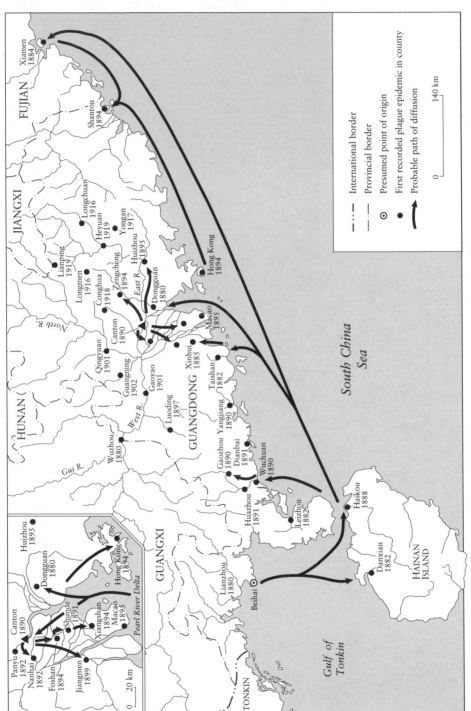

MAP 10 Plague diffusion along the South China coast, 1880–1919.

Legend:

- ––·–– International border
- ––·– Provincial border
- ⊙ Presumed point of origin
- ● First recorded plague epidemic in county
- → Probable path of diffusion

0   140 km

FUJIAN

Xiamen 1884

Shantou 1894

JIANGXI

Longchuan 1916

Heyuan 1919

Yongan 1917

Lianping 1919

Longmen 1916

Conghua 1918

Zengcheng 1894

Huizhou 1895

East R.

Dongguan 1880

Hong Kong 1894

North R.

Canton 1890

Qingyuan 1901

Guangning 1902

Macao 1895

HUNAN

Wuzhou 1880

Gui R.

West R.

Luoding 1897

Gaoyao 1901

Xinhui 1885

Taishan 1882

GUANGDONG

Yangjiang 1890

Gaozhou 1890

Dianbai 1891

Wuchuan 1890

Huazhou 1891

Leizhou 1882

Haikou 1888

South China Sea

Lianzhou 1880

Beihai ⊙

GUANGXI

Damxian 1882

HAINAN ISLAND

Gulf of Tonkin

TONKIN

Pearl River Delta

Huizhou 1895

Dongguan 1880

Hong Kong 1894

Canton 1890

Panyu 1892

Nanhai 1892

Shunde 1891

Xiangshan 1894

Macao 1895

Foshan 1894

Jiangmen 1899

0   20 km

TABLE 15

Recorded Epidemics Along the South China Coast, 1880–1919

Year	Location	Source consulted
1880	Lianzhou	*SYLXS* 1982: 1484
1880	Wuzhou	*SYLXS* 1982: 1684
1880	Dongguan	*SYLXS* 1982: 1606
1882	Leizhou	*SYLXS* 1982: 1557
1882	Danxian	*SYLXS* 1982: 1653
1882	Taishan	*SYLXS* 1982: 1593
1884	Xiamen	*SYLXS* 1982: 969
1885	Xinhui	*SYLXS* 1982: 1596
1888	Haikou	*SYLXS* 1982: 1658
1890	Wuchuan	*Wuchuanxian zhi* 1892 [1888], 10: 50b
1890	Gaozhou	Zheng Xiaoyan 1936 [1901]: preface
1890	Yangjiang	*SYLXS* 1982: 1568
1890	Canton (suburbs)	*SYLXS* 1982: 1606
1891	Huazhou	*SYLXS* 1982: 1568
1891	Dianbai	*SYLXS* 1982: 1581
1891	Shunde	*SYLXS* 1982: 1600
1892	Panyu	*Panyuxian xu zhi* 1931, 4: 7
1892	Nanhai	*SYLXS* 1982: 1594
1894	Canton	*Nanhaixian zhi* 1910, 2: 69a
1894	Hong Kong	Hong Kong Government, *Hong Kong Legislative Council Sessional Papers,* June 20, 1894
1894	Foshan	*SYLXS* 1982: 1596
1894	Xiangshan	*SYLXS* 1982: 1602
1894	Zengcheng	*SYLXS* 1982: 1608
1894	Shantou	*SYLXS* 1982: 1613
1895	Macao	*SYLXS* 1982: 1604
1895	Huizhou	*SYLXS* 1982: 1652
1897	Luoding	*SYLXS* 1982: 1582
1899	Jiangmen	*SYLXS* 1982: 1596
1901	Gaoyao	*(Xuantong) Gaoyaoxian zhi* 1938, 13: 45
1901	Qingyuan	*SYLXS* 1982: 1587
1902	Guangning	*SYLXS* 1982: 1590
1916	Longmen	*SYLXS* 1982: 1653
1916	Longchuan	*SYLXS* 1982: 1644
1917	Yongan	*SYLXS* 1982: 1647
1918	Conghua	*SYLXS* 1982: 1608
1919	Heyuan	*SYLXS* 1982: 1649
1919	Lianping	*SYLXS* 1982: 1650

NOTE: Only first recorded epidemics are listed. See *SYLXS* (1982: 1455–1680) for lists of plague epidemics in subsequent years.

northward to Shicheng county in 1877, and southward to Zhanjiang in 1879 (*Shichengxian zhi* 1931, 10: 34b; *SYLXS* 1982: 1490, 1570, and 1576).[17]

Plague continued to spread throughout the Leizhou Peninsula in the 1880's and early 1890's, affecting Leizhou prefecture in 1882 (*SYLXS* 1982: 1557). It also continued to be diffused along the inland route between Beihai and Wuzhou. Luchuan had an epidemic in 1888, and Rongxian in 1889 (ibid.: 1684). The disease moved farther east along the western Guangdong coastal route, reaching Gaozhou and Wuchuan in 1890 (ibid.: 1580, 1578; *Wuchuanxian zhi* 1892 [1888], 10: 50b) and Huazhou and Dianbai in 1891 (*SYLXS* 1982: 1568, 1581). Yangjiang had a plague outbreak in 1890 (ibid.: 1581). After this initial outbreak, plague disappeared in Yangjiang until 1897, but from that year until 1919 there were annual epidemics in the county.

The first recorded epidemic of plague on Hainan Island occurred in Danxian in 1882 (Lin Shiquan 1989: 100–101). (See Table 14 and Map 18.) The disease most likely spread to Hainan from the Leizhou Peninsula, which was experiencing an intense outbreak of plague in the same year (*SYLXS* 1982: 1557). The largest town on the island, Qiongshan and its port, Haikou, had outbreaks in 1888 (ibid.: 1658, 1660). Subsequent epidemics on Hainan appear either to have originated in these towns or to have spread directly across the strait from Leizhou.

Once plague became entrenched in western Guangdong, it was inevitable that it would reach the Pearl River Delta via the maritime transport network that stretched from Beihai up the South China coast. In the 1880's the disease spread to many of the small ports in central coastal Guangdong, and in the 1890's it reached Canton and Hong Kong (Table 15 and Map 19). From these two cities plague was rediffused not only throughout the Pearl River Delta and to inland communities along the many rivers that fed into the delta, but to international ports as well.

Conclusion

Plague was present in eastern Yunnan in the first two decades of the nineteenth century but only spilled over into Guangxi and western Guangdong during the 1860's. The fact that plague was largely contained within the Yungui region until the mid-nineteenth century suggests that some aspect of the spatial networks connecting the two regions was transformed during this period of time. One significant change was the development after 1830 of the Yunnan-Lingnan opium trade. The trade in Yunnan opium intensified the flow of goods and people between Yunnan and Guangxi and Guangdong, thereby enhancing the probability that plague would be carried from one region to the other.

The spread of plague was linked not only to greater interregional trade but to complex environmental and epidemiological factors as well. During the 1840's, the domestic opium trade was conducted primarily along the West River system, and passed through areas that are relatively inhospitable to the primary plague-carrier in southern China, the yellow-chested rat (*Rattus flavipectus*). Although plague was recorded periodically in districts along the West River in Guangxi, it never took hold there in the way that it did on the Leizhou Peninsula.

Between 1850 and 1860, large sections of the West River were impassable due to military blockades, active warfare, or the presence of hostile bandit groups or secret societies. Traders were forced to use other transport routes to and from Yunnan, routes that came to center on the town of Beihai. The area around Beihai and the entire Leizhou Peninsula make up an ecological area where the yellow-chested rat thrives (Ji Shuli 1988: 66). Between 1850 and 1870, the triangular zone stretching from southeastern Yunnan through Tonkin to Beihai and the Leizhou Peninsula was one in which the level of human movement was unusually high for a peripheral subregion (see Map 16). This intensified movement between southeastern Yunnan (where the disease was prevalent in the early 1860's) and the western Lingnan region allowed for the interregional spread of the disease. From the 1860's on, Beihai and the Leizhou Peninsula became a continued source of infection for towns in eastern and central Guangdong. The disease remained prevalent in communities on the Leizhou Peninsula throughout the twentieth century, and was only brought under control there after 1952.

CHAPTER 3

The Spatial Diffusion of Plague in the
Southeast Coast Macroregion, 1884-1949

IN CHAPTERS 1 and 2, I described the territorial spread of plague in the interior of China, focusing on the historical reasons for its movement first through Yunnan and then from Yunnan to the Lingnan region. I now shift from historical narrative to geographical analysis in order to discuss certain spatial and demographic dimensions of the nineteenth-century plague epidemics. This chapter describes the diffusion of plague within the boundaries of the Southeast Coast macroregion (Map 20).[1] It seeks to correlate the spread of the disease not only with the natural environment but with settlement patterns and the intraregional flows of goods and people as well. Contrary to much of the literature on the history of plague in other areas of the world, which holds that plague diffusion was erratic and unpredictable, I show that patterns of plague diffusion are discernible when the proper units of spatial analysis are chosen. In the Southeast Coast region, the disease spread largely within the boundaries of the regional-city trading systems demarcated by G. William Skinner (1985: 277). Although the fit is not perfect between Skinner's analytical framework and paths of diffusion (along the coast, plague crossed over the regional-city system boundaries drawn by Skinner), the concept of regional cities and their hinterlands allows for a more systematic assessment of plague diffusion than the simple "urban-rural" typology used in most historical studies on plague.

Concepts and Controversies

Concepts of Disease Diffusion

Medical geographers use the term "disease diffusion" to describe the process whereby infectious disease moves through space over time. Borrowing methods used by economic geographers to study the spatial diffusion of innovation, medical geographers describe three types of infectious disease diffusion (Pyle 1979: 137; Stock 1976: 2–4).[2] The first is relocation diffusion, which involves the jump of an infection from one region to another with no impact on the intervening territory. In the modern world, relocation diffusion typically occurs as the result of mechanized transport: contagious persons can travel far by air, rail, or highway. In preindustrial societies, relocation diffusion may have occurred where long-distance maritime, riverine, coach, or equestrian travel was possible. In the second pattern, urban-hierarchical diffusion, the degree to which the region is linked by efficient transportation networks is important. The rate of spread is greatest along major transportation arteries and between cities and their hinterlands. When an infectious disease is brought into a large city, it is likely to cascade from higher- to lower-order centers within the central-place hierarchy in a systematic fashion.

A third pattern is contact or expansion diffusion, where infectious disease spreads spatially and temporally outward from a central focus.[3] If no physiographic, cultural, or political barriers exist in an area and people can move about freely (as between village settlements on a plain or plateau), disease diffusion will occur in an unchanneled, wavelike pattern radiating out from the point of origin of infection through the rest of the region. Where there are natural channels (village settlements along a river or coastline), contact diffusion still occurs, but disease moves through or along the channel in a more linear way. The disease spreads to almost all communities in an area without regard for place in the urban hierarchy. In this instance an infection can move from rural areas to urban ones, or vice versa.

Diffusion processes are generally complex and typically display aspects of all three components. A contagious disease might be introduced into a major port city from abroad, move stepwise down through the urban hierarchy of the city's hinterland, and then spread radially outward to all communities in the region. In this scenario, a primary phase of relocation diffusion is followed by a secondary phase

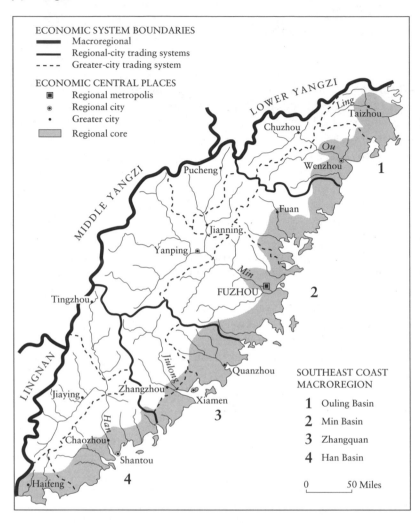

ECONOMIC SYSTEM BOUNDARIES
▬▬▬   Macroregional
▬▬▬   Regional-city trading systems
- - - -   Greater-city trading system

ECONOMIC CENTRAL PLACES
▣   Regional metropolis
◉   Regional city
•   Greater city
▨   Regional core

LOWER YANGZI

Ling
Taizhou
Chuzhou
Ou
Wenzhou   1

MIDDLE YANGZI

Pucheng

Fuan

Jianning

Yanping

Min

FUZHOU ▣   2

Tingzhou

LINGNAN

Jiulong

Quanzhou

SOUTHEAST COAST
MACROREGION

Jiaying   Zhangzhou
Xiamen
3

1 Ouling Basin
2 Min Basin
3 Zhangquan
4 Han Basin

Han

Chaozhou
Shantou

Haifeng   4

0   50 Miles

MAP 20. The Southeast Coast macroregion, ca. 1893. Adapted from
Skinner 1985: 277.

of urban-hierarchical diffusion and finally a tertiary phase of contact
diffusion. Conversely, if the disease is introduced into rural villages
first, it might follow a pattern of contact diffusion initially and only
then spread to larger cities (urban-hierarchical) or to other regions (relocation).[4]

Patterns of contagious disease diffusion have important implications for the rate of spread, the relative numbers of settlements infected in different subregions, and the demographic impact of a particular infection (Cliff et al. 1981: 26–27). People moving between rural villages on foot will spread the disease more slowly than people who are riding or driving longer distances. If disease is spread in a contact fashion alone, its relatively slow movement through an area means that, within a given period of time, fewer communities (and hence people) are affected. When a pure relocation pattern obtains, towns along the major transport routes may have outbreaks of disease in quick succession, but diffusion to rural villages may be minimal and the relative number of settlements affected throughout the region may be limited.[5]

The most rapid rate of spread and the highest number of infected settlements occur where an urban-hierarchical diffusion obtains. This pattern can be expected in a region with a highly commercialized agrarian economy, where transport is quite efficient but not yet mechanized, and where settlements are packed densely on the land. In such a region disease spreads rapidly between towns along the major transport corridors but does not bypass the rural hinterland entirely (as it might in an industrialized society, where relocation diffusion is more common).

The concepts of relocation, hierarchical, and contact diffusion can be readily integrated into a core-periphery regional systems framework. In regional peripheries, where transport is less efficient and the landscape more sparsely settled, diffusion should tend to follow a contact pattern because transportation networks are relatively underdeveloped. The peripheral nature of these settlements means that they are less likely to be in constant contact with urban centers of infection. Given the slower rate of spread of contact diffusion, the infection might fade away before reaching all settlements in an area. Because fewer people live in the periphery, absolute morbidity (and mortality) might be quite low, although the relative morbidity in those few villages affected might be quite high.

In mature agrarian societies, a mixed pattern of urban-hierarchical and contact diffusion is likely to occur in the regional core, where settlement density and transport efficiency are both high. The rate of the spread of disease is faster—and waves of diffusion occur more frequently—in the regional core than in the regional periphery because higher levels of commercialization and urbanization facilitate the rapid diffusion of disease between towns and from towns to villages. Large numbers of settlements, both urban and rural, are affected because villages in the regional core are linked to one another and to urban centers by intricate transport networks that have not yet been obviated by railroads or high-speed highways. Disease spreads along these transport networks from towns to villages in a "vertical" or urban-hierarchical fashion, and then between villages in a "horizontal" or contact manner, rapidly blanketing large areas. From these villages the disease can be reintroduced to towns and then rediffused through the urban hierarchy once again, returning to the villages in wave upon wave of disease. While absolute morbidity might be quite high in cities and towns, relative morbidity might be quite low because the total population in these settlements is so large. The highest relative morbidity should occur in rural villages situated in the regional core, near large towns or cities. In the suburban countryside nearly every village becomes infected again and again, and many people in each small settlement become sick.

These principles of spatial diffusion have been successfully applied not only to the geography of contagious diseases, such as influenza and measles, but also to infectious diseases, such as cholera (Cliff et al. 1981; Pyle 1969; Pyle 1986; Stock 1976). As a vectored disease, bubonic plague adds another layer of complexity to the diffusion process, but because the infective vectors of plague are typically carried from one place to another by humans, the basic principles of diffusion remain the same as those for directly contagious diseases. Scholars have long known that plague outbreaks tend to follow trade routes, and several historians have tried to describe the actual diffusion processes of bubonic plague in past epidemics. There has been considerable controversy over whether plague was predominantly an urban phenomenon or whether it occurred in nonurban settings as well. This problem is linked in turn to a debate over the levels of mortality caused by the fourteenth-century Black Death.

The Urban Versus Rural Nature of Plague

Beginning with the fourteenth-century Black Death, waves of plague swept over the European continent, significantly affecting its demographic, social, and economic structures. The importance of bubonic plague in European history has long been acknowledged, but there has been disagreement over the precise demographic effects of the disease. There are basically two schools of thought: those who believe that mortality due to plague was extraordinary, with perhaps as much as a third of Europe's population succumbing to the disease (Benedictow 1992: 204; Gottfried 1983: 77; Ziegler 1969: 230); and those who think that plague affected a much smaller fraction of the population (Shrewsbury 1970: 23–26; Twigg 1984).

Scholars on both sides of the debate have supported their estimates of the magnitude of plague mortality with geographical evidence. On the one hand are those who argue that plague could only occur in a highly urbanized region. This thesis has been most forcefully argued by J. F. D. Shrewsbury (1970: 23–26). Shrewsbury, a bacteriologist, contends that the epidemiology of plague is such that it requires a certain population density of rodent hosts to become epizootic in animals (and thus epidemic in humans), and that this density threshold was only reached in towns above a certain size. Moreover, Shrewsbury argues, plague was spread primarily between towns along well-established trade channels. Because some four-fifths of the English population in the fourteenth century lived in rural areas or small, out-of-the-way towns, Shrewsbury believes that most subregions of the country must have escaped the Black Death.

Shrewsbury's thesis that plague spreads primarily along major transport routes between larger towns has been supported by several empirical studies. Jean-Noël Biraben (1975, 1: 285–87) described the diffusion of the 1720–22 plague epidemic in southern France from Marseilles along the Mediterranean coast and up the Rhone River valley. He found that the disease moved from Marseilles to smaller cities and towns but only occasionally intruded into the countryside. This pattern of plague diffusion is similar to the one in seventeenth-century England described by Paul Slack (1985: 13, 86), where plague began in port cities, moved upriver from one major center of population to another, and only then diffused to smaller communities. Biraben and Slack's findings suggest that plague follows an "urban" pattern of diffusion, reaching primarily cities and towns located along maritime or riverine transport routes.

On the other side of the debate are those who demonstrate that plague was not confined to towns and cities but spread into rural areas far from major urban centers. In an analysis of plague mortality in Cilento, a rural district in southern Italy, Ole Jørgen Benedictow (1987: 407) found that not only did plague reach Cilento, but relative mortality was significantly higher in villages than it was in towns or cities. Cilento was linked by overland transport to the port of Naples but had neither good harbors of its own nor any important communications lines (ibid.: 413–15). Yet, between 1656 and 1670, plague reached every community in the area, spreading to even the smallest settlements.

In two studies of plague epidemics in Switzerland between 1628 and 1629, Edward Eckert (1978, 1982) found a pattern similar to that described by Benedictow. Eckert's studies focus on four cantons in the northern part of Switzerland. The study area contains low-lying mountains and foothills and an extensive plateau of flat or rolling farmland. In the seventeenth century it was heavily populated but predominantly rural, with inhabitants broadly dispersed among a large number of farming communities. There were no cities close by. Nonetheless, plague outbreaks were distributed broadly over the plateau, and two-thirds of all communities suffered severe loss of life during the epidemic. Benedictow and Eckert's studies point to a "rural" pattern of plague diffusion whereby a large number of communities are affected regardless of their size.

Although each of these authors refers in passing to the broader geographical context in which these epidemics occurred, none attempts to use a functionally integrated region as his unit of analysis. Clearly, they are describing different parts of interrelated regional systems. Slack and Biraben are describing two maritime cities in the regional core, whereas Benedictow and Eckert are focusing on rural areas in the hinterland of such cities. Biraben and Slack describe the urban-hierarchical diffusion of plague in suburban villages near Marseilles and London but neglect to examine the diffusion of the disease farther from these cities. Benedictow acknowledges that the rural epidemics had their origins in Naples but fails to link the two in any systematic way. Eckert is more sensitive to a regional approach, mentioning that the Swiss epidemics originated in towns on the North Sea coast (in Holland) and spread down the Rhine River corridor. Nonetheless, his analysis focuses primarily on diffusion processes in rural areas without reference to their urban origins. In light of the work done by Eckert and Benedictow, Slack and Biraben's implicit assumption that plague was predominantly an urban phenomenon is no longer convincing. Eckert and Benedictow, however, have not been able to show that plague spread through rural areas without having been first imported from an urban center. The failure of each of these four authors to ground his findings in a broader regional context gives rise to the particular "urban" and "rural" patterns of diffusion each describes, none of which is satisfactory.

Observed Patterns of Plague Diffusion in China

The concepts of "urban" and "rural" plague can be found not only in historical writing on plague but in much of the modern epidemiological literature as well. R. Pollitzer (1954: 490–91), an epidemiologist who conducted research on plague in China in the 1930's, used an urban-rural typology to describe the process of plague diffusion he observed in Fujian province. "Urban" plague diffusion typically occurred after the disease appeared in a major seaport. This was followed by the spread of the infection to inland towns connected to the port by major traffic routes. Pollitzer observed that, when a new county became infected by plague, the disease usually invaded the county capital or the market town first and then spread to surrounding villages. He also noted that the range and speed of diffusion depended on the commercial importance of the urban center and its location in the transport network. From higher-order centers plague was distributed to a wide area in a rapid fashion; from lower-order centers it moved more slowly and spread to a smaller area. When plague followed an urban pattern of diffusion, larger villages and those situated near the major lines of communication were more severely affected than were more peripheral villages, and the proportion of small villages that remained free of infection was quite high.

The "rural" pattern Pollitzer describes usually appeared only secondarily, after the disease was imported into rural villages from the closest market town: plague then spread horizontally from one village to another in a random fashion. During the rural phase, the disease could also spread from a village back to the market town or county capital from which it had been introduced, and from there be redistributed to other villages in the area. This resulted in a higher proportion of small villages being affected than when plague followed an urban pattern of diffusion, even though the path of the disease was erratic and not all villages had epidemics in a given year. Pollitzer describes this as "area-wide endemicity," by which he means that the entire area had annual plague outbreaks for a number of years, although no one village in the area had the disease for more than one or two seasons. Each village was affected in turn, and plague might return to a village where it had been absent for some years.

William Landauer, another epidemiologist, studied plague diffusion on Hainan Island (in Guangdong province; see Chapter 2) in the 1930's (Pollitzer 1954: 496). Landauer also found that plague epidemics on

Hainan moved through two distinct phases. The towns were infected first, but after a number of violent epidemics, the disease gradually died out. The second stage (which did not always occur) consisted of the spread of the disease into the countryside. Epidemics in rural villages tended to be sporadic and small (on average about ten people per village affected), but the disease continued to be "endemic" in rural areas, and very often towns that had been free of the disease for a number of years were reinfected from the villages.

Although Pollitzer and Landauer termed these two patterns "urban" and "rural" plague, they are in essence describing two phases of the same epidemic: a primary phase of urban-hierarchical diffusion from city to town to village (urban plague), followed by a secondary phase of contact diffusion between villages (rural plague). Landauer's observations on Hainan Island corroborate Pollitzer's assessment that plague first followed an urban-hierarchical pattern and only then moved into a contact pattern between villages. Despite their use of the terms "urban" and "rural," their descriptions make it clear that diffusion occurred systematically through a functionally integrated region.

Pollitzer and Landauer observed plague diffusion in areas of China where areawide endemicity had already been achieved. By the 1930's, when they made their studies, plague was entrenched in coastal Fujian and on Hainan Island. To get a clearer picture of how the disease was diffused through southeastern China, it is necessary to focus on the last two decades of the nineteenth century, when the modern pandemic first reached these areas.

The Diffusion of Plague in the Southeast Coast Region

The Southeast Coast Macroregion

Fujian province is part of the broader Southeast Coast macroregion (Skinner 1985: 277). The region is defined by several rivers that flow east from the Wuyi Mountains to the coast. Within the macroregion are four major subregional systems, all in the drainage basins of these rivers: the Ou River, with the delta city of Wenzhou (located in Zhejiang province) as regional city; the Min River Basin, dominated by the regional metropolis of Fuzhou (Foochow); the Jiulong River Basin, which was centered on Xiamen (Amoy) and which included the greater cities of Zhangzhou and Quanzhou (the Zhangquan subregion); and the Han River in the northeastern corner of Guangdong province, with the regional city of Shantou (Swatow) as its economic center. In the nineteenth century Taiwan was also part of the regional system, Tainan being the largest city on the island. Within each of the four regional-city trading systems on the mainland were subregions defined by greater cities and their hinterlands (see Map 20).

The core-periphery structure of the Southeast Coast region basically followed its physiographic structure. There is little low-lying land around the major cities of the southeast, most of which are situated on the coast. The coastal lowlands quickly give way to a mountainous interior characterized by deep, narrow, isolated valleys. With high levels of population density and urban concentration, the area along the coast formed the core of the regional system; the periphery stretched into the mountains.

In the late nineteenth century, transport through the region moved primarily along the coast or on the rivers (Tōa Dōbunkai 1919, 14: 353–424). There was a coastal road connecting Wenzhou with Chaozhou, but trade and transport between cities in the core took place for the most part via coastal junk traffic. Most of the rivers could be used only by small junks or bamboo rafts that were hauled upstream by trackers through narrow valleys leading to poor, peripheral towns. Two exceptions were the area along the upper reaches of the Min River and the northern branch of the Jiulong River, both of which were navigable by larger boats. Yanping, located upriver from Fuzhou, served as the center for towns along the many rivers that converged to form the Min River. The northern branch of the Jiulong River in the southern part of Fujian could also be navigated upstream.

The Ecology of Plague in the Southeast Coast Region

Areas of the Southeast Coast region, particularly southern Fujian, are part of the Commensal Rat Plague Focus that now dots southern China (Ji Shuli 1988: 64). There are four plague-carrying rodents in the region: *Rattus flavipectus* (the yellow-chested rat), *Rattus norvegicus* (the common brown rat), *Mus musculus* (the common house mouse), and *Suncus murinus* (the house shrew). Researchers have determined that the yellow-chested rat and the common brown rat are the two most effective carriers of plague in the region, with the former being the most numerous. In a study conducted in the 1950's, *Rattus norvegicus* represented only 8 percent of all rodents caught in the southern part of Fujian province (the area around Xiamen), while *Rattus flavi-*

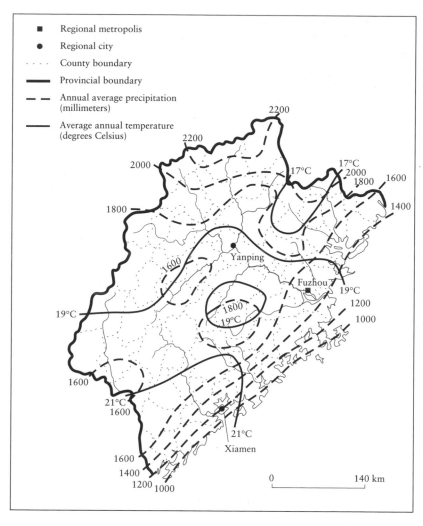

■   Regional metropolis

●   Regional city

· · · ·   County boundary

──   Provincial boundary

─ ─   Annual average precipitation
       (millimeters)

──   Average annual temperature
       (degrees Celsius)

MAP 21. Annual precipitation and average temperatures in Fujian. Adapted from *SYLXS* 1982, 2: 942.

pectus represented about 58 percent. In the northern part of Fujian, around Fuzhou, *Rattus norvegicus* represented about 18 percent of all trapped rodents, and *Rattus flavipectus* represented about 40 percent.[6] There are twenty-five types of fleas in the Southeast Coast region, but the most important for plague transmission is the Asiatic rat flea

(*Xenopsylla cheopis*), which is commonly found on both the *Rattus flavi-pectus* and the *Rattus norvegicus*. In the southern part of Fujian, this flea represented 75 percent of fleas found on captured commensal rodents (ibid.: 194).

Southern and northern Fujian (Minnan and Minbei) have different plague seasons. Plague appears in the south in April, May, June, and July (with July being the high point); in the north it appears in March and April, and then again in August, September, and October. The seasonality of the disease is related to climate and the effect of climate on *Xenopsylla cheopis* fleas (Map 21). Throughout Fujian, the bubonic form of plague is the most prevalent. Between 1950 and 1952, it represented 95 percent of all cases; the pneumonic form appeared in only 4 percent of all documented cases. Other types of plague were hardly seen.

Over the course of the twentieth century, plague epidemics in the region have appeared most frequently along the coastal area around Xiamen (Map 22). This is partially because the climate along the coast is warm enough and humid enough for both the *Rattus flavipectus* rodent and the *Xenopsylla cheopis* flea to thrive (*SYLXS* 1982: 952). However, climatic factors alone cannot account for the spatial distribution of these frequent plague outbreaks. Features of human geography must also be considered, which requires in turn that plague outbreaks in Fujian be placed in the proper analytical framework—namely, that of the regional-city systems of the Southeast Coast macroregion.

The Spread of Plague in the Regional-City Systems of the Southeast Coast

The spread of plague in the Southeast Coast macroregion generally took place within the boundaries of four regional-city trading systems and their hinterlands.[7] Map 23 provides an overview of plague diffusion through the Xiamen, Fuzhou, Yanping, and Shantou regional-city trading systems.[8] The disease arrived in Xiamen in 1884 (year 1), spread northward along the coast toward Fuzhou (in 1890, or year 7), inland along the two branches of the Jiulong River, and southward along the coast. From Fuzhou, plague spread south to coastal communities, up the Min River to interior cities and towns, and eventually to the northern coastal area. The disease appeared in Shantou in 1894 (year 11) and diffused rapidly through the Han River Basin, both up the Han River and along the coast. In 1900 (year 17) plague moved from Fuzhou up the Min River to Yanping, from which it diffused slowly to counties in the far interior.

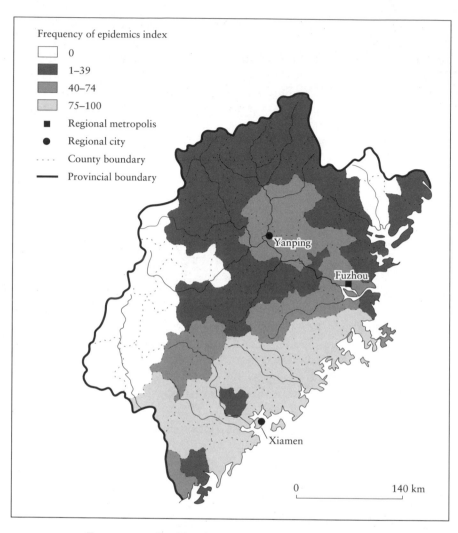

MAP 22. Frequency of epidemics in Fujian, by county, 1884–1952. Adapted from *SYLXS* 1982, 2: 942. The occurrence of epidemics by county was only recorded annually. The raw score on which the index for each county is based was computed by giving each county a score of 1 for each year in which an epidemic was recorded and 0 for each year in which no epidemic was recorded there.

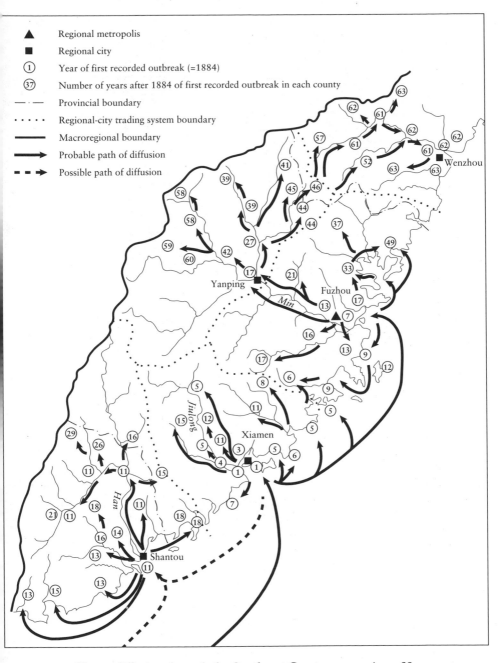

MAP 23. Plague diffusion through the Southeast Coast macroregion, 1884–1949.

TABLE 16
Recorded Plague Epidemics in the Xiamen Regional-City Trading System, 1884–98

Year	Location	Source consulted
1884	Xiamen	*SYLXS* 1982: 969
1884	Haicheng	*SYLXS* 1982: 977
1886	Tongan	*SYLXS* 1982: 988
1887	Longxi	*SYLXS* 1982: 980
1888	Nan'an	*SYLXS* 1982: 1015
1888	Huian	*SYLXS* 1982: 1044
1888	Nanjing	*SYLXS* 1982: 1150
1888	Zhangping	*SYLXS* 1982: 1157
1889	Jinjiang	*SYLXS* 1982: 1162
1890	Zhangpu	*SYLXS* 1982: 1220
1891	Yongchun	*SYLXS* 1982: 1230
1894	Anxi	*SYLXS* 1982: 1282
1894	Changtai	*SYLXS* 1982: 1294
1895	Hua'an	*SYLXS* 1982: 1305
1898	Longyan	*SYLXS* 1982: 1342

NOTE: Only first recorded epidemics are listed. See *SYLXS* (1982: 931–1454) for lists of plague epidemics that occurred in subsequent years.

Three of these regional-city trading systems, Xiamen, Shantou, and Fuzhou, were situated in the regional core of the Southeast Coast macroregion. Plague diffusion in these subregions was quite rapid, with many counties affected within a few years of the initial outbreak in Xiamen. Large numbers of both towns and villages were affected, and the estimated plague mortality (absolute number of deaths due to plague) was quite high (*SYLXS* 1982, 2: 931–1454). In contrast, plague diffusion through the more peripherally located Yanping regional-city trading system was relatively slow and sporadic, the total number of communities affected was small, and the estimated number of plague deaths rather low. The spatial pattern of plague diffusion through these four subregions thus supports the hypothesis that plague mortality is correlated to location in the core-periphery regional structure. The next sections discuss these patterns in greater detail.[9]

Xiamen and Its Hinterland.   The first recorded appearance of plague in the Southeast Coast region occurred in Xiamen in 1884 (*SYLXS* 1982: 969). (See Table 16.) The disease may have been imported into Xiamen from Danxian on Hainan Island in Guangdong province, which had experienced its first outbreak two years before. Hainan and Xiamen had very strong economic and cultural ties because many of the Hainanese had originally emigrated from the area around Xiamen (Skinner 1957:

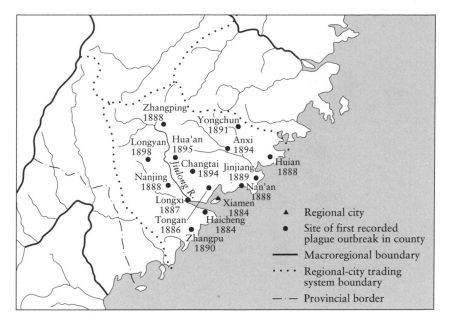

MAP 24. Plague diffusion through the Xiamen regional-city trading system.

39). The county of Haicheng, located on the mainland directly across from Xiamen Island, also had a plague outbreak in 1884 (*SYLXS* 1982: 977). As shown in Table 16 and Map 24, plague was diffused relatively quickly from Xiamen to coastal counties, such as Tongan and Longxi, which were in direct communication with the port. Plague also spread relatively rapidly up the Jiulong River and inland from the coast.

Figure 1 shows estimated numbers of deaths due to plague from 1884 to 1949 for counties lying within the Xiamen regional-city trading system.[10] After the 1884 introduction of the disease into Xiamen, few deaths from plague were reported in the regional-city system until 1887, when there seems to have been a sharp rise in such fatalities.[11] Two sharp peaks occurred in 1896 and 1899, years in which close to thirty thousand people reportedly died from plague. After 1900 the numbers of deaths due to plague tapered off, and after 1909 the number remained below ten thousand per year until the 1940's.

In Figure 2 the numbers of villages (*cun*) affected by plague in the Xiamen regional-city trading system are plotted over time.[12] This num-

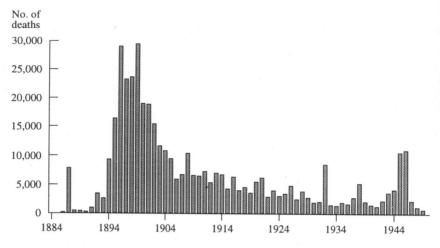

FIG. 1. Estimated deaths due to plague in the Xiamen regional-city trading system, 1884–1949. Derived from *SYLXS* 1982, 2: 931–1454.

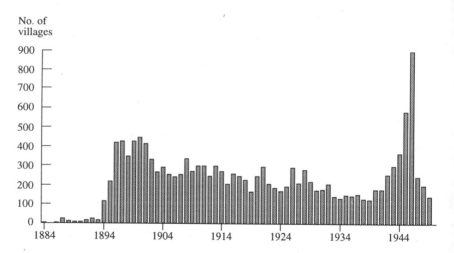

FIG. 2. Number of villages with plague outbreaks in the Xiamen regional-city trading system, 1884–1949. Derived from *SYLXS* 1982, 2: 931–1454.

ber first peaked in 1900, when some four hundred fifty villages had outbreaks of plague. There was then a gradual diminution in the number of villages where plague appeared, a trend that continued into the 1930's. The relative flatness of the curve after 1902 suggests that area-wide endemicity, as described by Pollitzer, had been achieved by that time. Both the numbers of reported plague deaths and the numbers of

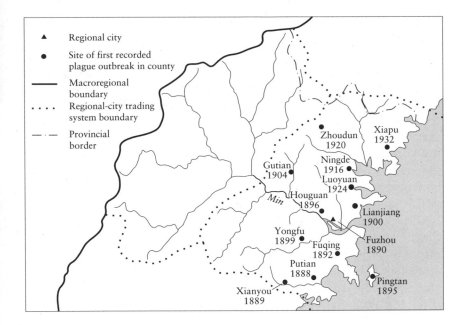

MAP 25. Plague diffusion through the Fuzhou regional-city trading system.

TABLE 17

Recorded Plague Epidemics in the Fuzhou Regional-City Trading System, 1888–1932

Year	Location	Source consulted
1888	Putian	*SYLXS* 1982: 1095
1889	Xianyou	*SYLXS* 1982: 1199
1890	Fuzhou	*SYLXS* 1982: 959
1892	Fuqing	*SYLXS* 1982: 1244
1895	Pingtan	*SYLXS* 1982: 1309
1896	Houguan	*SYLXS* 1982: 1317
1899	Yongfu	*SYLXS* 1982: 1368
1900	Lianjiang	*SYLXS* 1982: 1377
1904	Gutian	*SYLXS* 1982: 1388
1916	Ningde	*SYLXS* 1982: 1407
1920	Zhoudun	*SYLXS* 1982: 1409
1924	Luoyuan	*SYLXS* 1982: 1415
1932	Xiapu	*SYLXS* 1982: 1432

NOTE: Only first recorded epidemics are listed. See *SYLXS* (1982: 931–1454) for lists of plague epidemics in subsequent years.

villages affected increased during the 1940's, undoubtedly as a result of wartime hardships.

Fuzhou and Its Hinterland.   Along the coast, particularly in the very heavily settled counties lying between Xiamen and Fuzhou (see Map 22), the land-based regional-city trading system was less important in the diffusion of the disease than was the maritime transport network that linked coastal communities. Fishing vessels and small junks were not constrained by the physiographic barriers that bound marketing systems on land, and they moved freely up and down the Fujian coast between Xiamen and Fuzhou. This accounts for the one instance in which plague diffusion transcended the boundaries of regional-city trading systems in the Southeast Coast region (Map 25 and Table 17).[13] Plague appears to have spread to Putian and Xianyou from Xiamen rather than from Fuzhou, even though these two counties are situated in Fuzhou's hinterland. The disease did not appear in Fuzhou until 1890 (*SYLXS* 1982: 959). From there it diffused rapidly to communities lying along the Min River. Counties in the northeastern quadrant of Fuzhou's hinterland (Luoyuan, Ningde, Zhoudun, and Xiapu) were only affected much later.

Figure 3 shows estimated numbers of deaths due to plague in the Fuzhou regional-city trading system between 1888 and 1949. The curve is similar to the one for the Xiamen regional-city trading system (see Figure 1). A sharp rise in the estimated numbers of people dying from plague occurred in 1898 (when some twelve thousand deaths were reported) and in 1902 (some twenty-five thousand deaths). Then there was a decline to below five thousand annually. Most of these deaths occurred in the coastal counties of Putian, Xianyou, Fuqing, and Pingtan. The number of villages affected (shown in Figure 4) demonstrates a similar pattern: a sharp increase in 1898 and 1902, followed by a leveling off between 1904 and 1943, and a rise during the Second World War. Again, the flatness of the curve after 1902 suggests that endemicity had been achieved by that time, and that few new villages were affected until the 1940's.

Shantou and Its Hinterland.   The regional city of Shantou had its first recorded outbreak of plague in 1894 (Cousland 1896: 23–24; *SYLXS* 1982: 1614). (See Table 18 and Map 26.)[14] It is not clear whether the disease spread to Shantou from Xiamen or from Canton and Hong Kong: both areas were suffering a major outbreak of plague that year. In any event, once the disease appeared in Shantou, it moved rapidly both

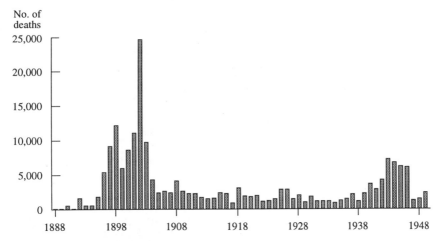

FIG. 3. Estimated deaths due to plague in the Fuzhou regional-city trading system, 1888–1949. Derived from *SYLXS* 1982, 2: 931–1454.

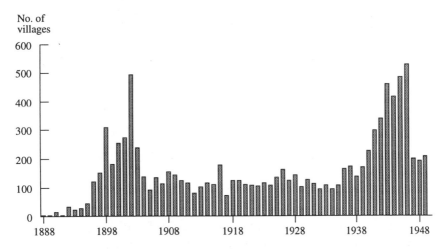

FIG. 4. Number of villages with plague outbreaks in the Fuzhou regional-city trading system, 1888–1949. Derived from *SYLXS* 1982, 2: 931–1454.

TABLE 18

Recorded Plague Epidemics in the Shantou Regional-City Trading System,
1894–1912

Year	Location	Source consulted
1894	Shantou	*SYLXS* 1982: 1614
1894	Meizhou	*SYLXS* 1982: 1623
1894	Xingning	*SYLXS* 1982: 1632
1894	Raoping	*SYLXS* 1982: 1618
1894	Dapu	*SYLXS* 1982: 1620
1896	Puning	*SYLXS* 1982: 1627
1896	Huilai	*SYLXS* 1982: 1632
1896	Haifeng	*SYLXS* 1982: 1648
1897	Chaoyang	*SYLXS* 1982: 1229
1898	Lufeng	*SYLXS* 1982: 1643
1899	Jieyang	*SYLXS* 1982: 1626
1899	Yongding	*SYLXS* 1982: 1350
1901	Fengshun	*SYLXS* 1982: 1624
1901	Dongshan	*SYLXS* 1982: 1380
1901	Yunxiao	*SYLXS* 1982: 1384
1901	Zhaoan	*SYLXS* 1982: 1385
1904	Wuhua	*SYLXS* 1982: 1642
1909	Zhenping	*SYLXS* 1982: 1621
1912	Pingyuan	*SYLXS* 1982: 1621

NOTE: Only first recorded epidemics are listed. See *SYLXS* (1982: 931–1454) for lists of plague epidemics in subsequent years.

along the coast and in the interior of the Han River Basin. Throughout the 1890's and into the first two decades of the twentieth century, plague continued to appear in Shantou and interior counties, and was particularly prevalent in Xingning county. It eventually spread to more peripheral counties in the subregion.

Yanping and Its Hinterland.   The Yanping prefectural seat is located at the conjuncture of three rivers that form the Min River.[15] In the nineteenth century it served as the regional city for the upper Min River Basin. The pattern of diffusion from Yanping to towns in its hinterland is quite clear-cut: plague came rather slowly to the Yanping subregion, outbreaks being limited in number and sporadic in periodicity (Table 19 and Map 27). Yanping itself had its first outbreak of plague in 1900, clearly as the consequence of the movement of goods and people up the Min River (*SYLXS* 1982: 1371). Following the 1900–1902 epidemic, plague did not reappear in Yanping until 1911, after a 1910 outbreak in Jian'an. The disease spread to communities farther upriver only in the 1920's. Counties located in the far interior were not affected until the 1940's.

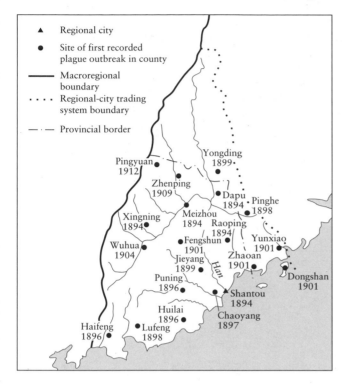

▲ Regional city

● Site of first recorded
   plague outbreak in county

── Macroregional
    boundary

· · · · Regional-city trading
        system boundary

— · — Provincial border

Pingyuan● 1912

Yongding 1899●

Zhenping 1909●

Dapu 1894● Pinghe ●1898

Xingning 1894●

Meizhou 1894 Raoping 1894

Wuhua 1904●

Fengshun ●1901

Yunxiao 1901●

Zhaoan 1901●

Jieyang 1899●

Puning 1896●

Dongshan 1901

Shantou 1894▲

Huilai 1896●

Haifeng 1896/●

Lufeng ●1898

Chaoyang 1897

Han

MAP 26. Plague diffusion through the Shantou regional-city trading system.

The estimated numbers of deaths due to plague and villages where the disease appeared in the Yanping regional-city trading system are plotted in Figures 5 and 6. Plague took a long time to spread to and within the Yanping subregion: the peak of the epidemic did not occur until 1930, when some three thousand people in the subregion reportedly died of the disease. Throughout the first decades of the twentieth century, the number of villages affected was consistently below 110; the high point of 109 villages did not occur until 1945 (see Figure 6).

In Figure 7 I have indexed the estimated numbers of deaths due to plague in each of the three systems in order to highlight the differences between plague diffusion in the regional-city system of Yanping on the one hand and of Xiamen and Fuzhou on the other. The epidemic curves of the Xiamen and Fuzhou regional-city trading systems are similar in shape, the only significant difference being a slight time lag for the Fuzhou epidemics. Plague spread rapidly through these

TABLE 19
Recorded Plague Epidemics in the Yanping Regional-City Trading System,
1900–1943

Year	Location	Source consulted
1900	Yanping	*SYLXS* 1982: 1371
1910	Jian'an	*SYLXS* 1982: 1393
1922	Jianyang	*SYLXS* 1982: 1412
1922	Chongan	*SYLXS* 1982: 1414
1924	Pucheng	*SYLXS* 1982: 1417
1925	Shunchang	*SYLXS* 1982: 1419
1927	Zhenghe	*SYLXS* 1982: 1419
1927	Pingnan	*SYLXS* 1982: 1426
1928	Songxi	*SYLXS* 1982: 1427
1941	Shaowu	*SYLXS* 1982: 1437
1941	Guangze	*SYLXS* 1982: 1437
1942	Taining	*SYLXS* 1982: 1439
1943	Jiangle	*SYLXS* 1982: 1440

NOTE: Only first recorded epidemics are listed. See *SYLXS* (1982: 931–1454) for lists of plague epidemics in subsequent years.

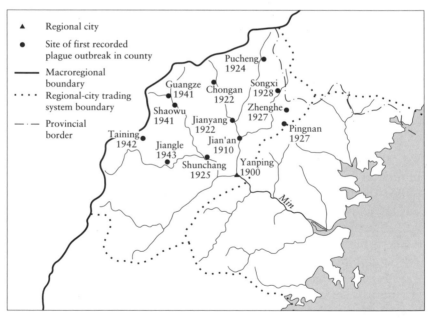

MAP 27. Plague diffusion through the Yanping regional-city trading system.

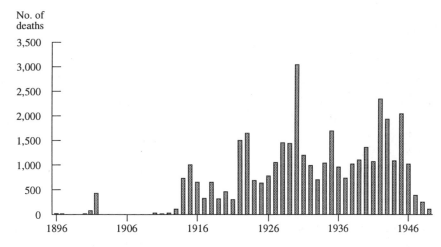

FIG. 5. Estimated deaths due to plague in the Yanping regional-city trading system, 1896–1949. Derived from *SYLXS* 1982, 2: 931–1454.

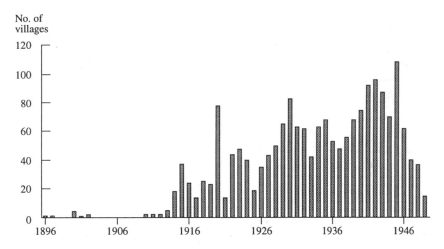

FIG. 6. Number of villages with plague outbreaks in the Yanping regional-city trading system, 1896–1949. Derived from *SYLXS* 1982, 2: 931–1454.

subregions and caused large numbers of deaths. In contrast, the Yanping curve shows a slow process of diffusion and very low numbers of deaths relative to the other two subregions.

The slow pattern of plague diffusion in the Yanping regional-city trading system was a consequence of its more peripheral location

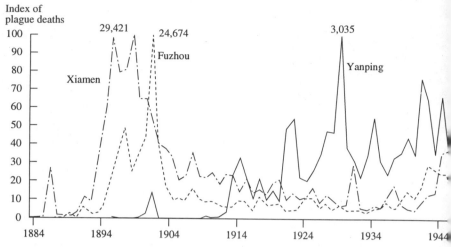

FIG. 7. Comparison of epidemic curves of estimated plague deaths in three regional-city trading systems of the Southeast Coast macroregion, 1884–1949. Derived from *SYLXS* 1982, 2: 931–1454. (Year with highest number of deaths equals 100.)

in the Southeast Coast macroregion. Situated in the far interior of a mountainous subregion, Yanping had much lower population densities than the subregions located on the coast, each of which contained counties that were heavily populated, highly urbanized and commercialized, and that had highly efficient riverine and maritime transport. In the more peripheral interior, plague epidemics were both less common than they were along the coast and seemingly less devastating in terms of absolute mortality.

Conclusion

Historians and epidemiologists who have studied plague have long been concerned with the process of its diffusion through space because they recognize that analysis of plague's demographic and social impact requires a prior knowledge of its geographical distribution and the territorial pattern of its spread. Although the broad patterns of plague diffusion between settlements have long been discerned (along major communications routes, between major towns, from towns to villages or vice versa, and horizontally between villages), a systematic framework for analyzing these patterns has been lacking. Previous studies of plague diffusion have failed to delineate the boundaries of functionally integrated regions within which the disease spread. Instead, much of the literature on plague uses an urban-rural typology to describe the geographical diffusion of the disease. Comparisons are often made between urban and rural areas without any discussion of the relationship between the two. This has led to much confusion and has given rise to the assumption that there is an "inexplicable randomness" in the spread of the disease (Slack 1985: 108).

The fundamental purpose of this chapter has been to suggest that there are no uniquely "urban" or "rural" patterns of plague diffusion but, rather, complex and overlapping diffusion processes that occur within and between functionally defined regions. The first step has been to determine the proper units of spatial analysis. In the case of the Southeast Coast macroregion, the regional-city trading system proved to be the area through which plague spread. The physiographic boundaries of the regional-city trading system effectively slowed the frequent flow of goods, people, and plague across subregional borders. The disease did spread across systemic boundaries along the coast between Xiamen and Fuzhou because maritime traffic was not inhibited by the physical barriers found on land. Nonetheless, most plague diffusion occurred within the borders of those regional-city trading systems where ecological conditions allowed the disease to take hold.

This analysis is preliminary, and it is too soon to conclude that the regional-city trading system is the most relevant unit to use in analyzing plague diffusion elsewhere. To determine its general utility, similar studies would have to be conducted for other regions of China, such as those discussed in the first two chapters. Unfortunately, the kind of information used to analyze plague diffusion in the Southeast Coast region is simply not available for the Lingnan and Yungui regions, and therefore such comparisons are not possible.

At the beginning of this chapter I hypothesized that location in the core-periphery structure of a region might affect the particular pattern of disease diffusion that obtained there, and consequently the morbidity (and mortality) rates of a subregion. I argued that a mixed pattern of urban-hierarchical and contact diffusion should be present in the regional core, while a contact pattern alone should obtain in the regional periphery. A more finely grained study of plague diffusion in particular subregions is needed to determine whether or not this was the case—analysis that is not possible with the available data.

A rough comparison of plague diffusion through the three regional-city trading systems has shown that settlements situated in two coastal areas (Xiamen and Fuzhou) had far more intense and frequent episodes of plague than did the regionally more peripheral Yanping area. Because reliable population figures are not available, relative plague morbidity and mortality rates cannot be calculated. Diffusion patterns can nonetheless serve as a proxy indicator of plague's relative effects on these different subregions. As predicted, areas with the greatest number of settlements affected by plague (both urban and rural) and the highest estimated numbers of deaths due to plague were those in the regional core. In the Xiamen and Fuzhou systems, a mixed pattern of urban-hierarchical and contact diffusion may well explain why the disease circulated so rapidly, spread to many small villages as well as to large towns, and appeared year after year in so many communities.

The regional systems approach, which G. William Skinner and others have successfully used to analyze China's historical economic and social geography, is thus also helpful when studying the geographical diffusion of plague. When functional regions are used — rather than uniform categories such as "urban" or "rural" — plague is seen to spread across the landscape in ways that are complex and varied, to be sure, but not random and unpredictable. Were social scientists and historians interested in the differential effects of plague on city and countryside to ground their analyses in a regional systems framework, they might find not only that diffusion processes vary systematically through the core and periphery structures of functionally integrated regions, but that the disease's demographic impact does as well.

Reliable statistics that would allow for analysis of plague's demographic effects on nineteenth-century China are unavailable (see Appendixes). I suspect that, although plague may have devastated local communities, its overall impact on China's large population was barely perceptible. As Walter Lay, the commissioner of customs in Fuzhou between 1892 and 1901, wrote, "The plague was very prevalent throughout the summer months of the year [1901], reaching, it is said, 800 a day. The population is, however, so large, that a loss of 800 a day seems really quite infinitesimal" (Inspectorate General, *Decennial Reports* 1892–1901: 106).

The fact that plague may not have had any long-lasting demographic effects does not mean that it left no imprint on Chinese society. As our own contemporary experience with AIDS has reminded us, the social and psychological impact of an epidemic cannot be measured solely by the absolute number of deaths it causes or its effects on overall mortality. Ultimately, the measure of the social effects of bubonic plague can be seen in the varied ways the Chinese tried to cope with the crisis. As the next chapter will show, nineteenth-century Chinese society had a number of medical, religious, and administrative responses to epidemic plague. Interesting in their own right, these responses also provide eloquent testimony to the pain and suffering the disease brought to those communities confronted by it.

CHAPTER 4

Nineteenth-Century Chinese Medical, Religious, and Administrative Responses to Plague

THE SOCIAL response of any community to the crisis posed by epidemic plague is conditioned by beliefs about the etiology of the disease. In Christian Europe, explanations of the disease's origins were generally multilayered and included both natural and supernatural causes. Plague was seen as "Divine Will" as well as the consequence of naturally occurring, contagious miasmas (Park 1993: 614–15; Slack 1988: 436–40). Both interpretations served as rationalizations for the segregation of plague victims and the quarantine of stricken communities. The idea that plague was caused by miasmal vapors was also present in the Islamic Middle East, where this naturalistic interpretation was overlaid with the religious belief that plague was a mercy from God. People in plague-stricken areas were urged by Islamic theologians not to flee but to stay and welcome their martyrdom (Dols 1977: 109).

In nineteenth-century China—as earlier, in Europe and the Middle East—there were multiple and conflicting explanations of the disease, ranging from classical medical interpretations to beliefs about its ghostly origins. Seemingly contradictory ideas about the nature of plague were often held simultaneously by the same person. These beliefs inspired a variety of responses on both the individual and communal level. The families of the afflicted might visit a doctor and consult a spirit medium. Communities carried out neighborhood cleanup campaigns along with ritualistic exorcisms. Officials provided charitable medical relief and appealed to local plague gods. To understand the diverse ways the Chinese responded to plague in the nineteenth century and to compare these responses to those of preindustrial Europe and the Middle East, it is necessary first to discuss varying medical interpretations of plague and religious beliefs about its origins.

Classical Chinese Medical Interpretations of Plague

The disease that biomedicine terms "plague" did not exist in the classical Chinese medical lexicon.[1] Nineteenth-century Chinese medical practitioners identified plague as a type of exogenous heat illness, a set of disorders thought to be caused by "external illness factors" (*wai yin*) and to have fevers and hot sensations as their primary symptoms (Sivin 1987: 84). This broad category generally encompassed most acute febrile illnesses classified by biomedicine as "infectious disease" but was not synonymous with that group. Indeed, the very notion of disease is not very useful when discussing classical Chinese medical discourse. Unlike biomedicine, which rests on the assumption that motion and change are abnormal and need to be explained, Chinese medicine begins with the proposition that transformation is intrinsic to existence (Farquhar 1994: 24–28). Since there are no fixed essences in Chinese medical thought, the anatomical structures, reductive disease categories, and cause-and-effect relationships of biomedicine do not obtain. Chinese doctors do not think of the body as a stable form or of illness as an identifiable entity; rather, they view both physiology and pathology as constantly evolving processes. The highly contingent nature of any illness precludes assigning it to a rigid category in a taxonomy of disease.

This is not to suggest that Chinese physicians dispense with modes of classification altogether. The task of any Chinese medical doctor is to discern patterns in a patient's symptoms (*zheng*1) that can be specified as syndromes (*zheng*2) and then acted on with drug therapy (ibid.: 36–37). Because physicians classify dynamic forms (symptoms) rather than stable entities (diseases), the process of syndrome differentiation and treatment determination (*bianzheng lunzhi*) produces alternative diagnoses and strategies for treatment depending on the particular diagnostic method employed.

Several distinct diagnostic techniques, each associated with a particular school of thought, developed over the many centuries of classical Chinese medical practice.[2] By the nineteenth century there were two dominant doctrines concerned primarily with exogenous heat illnesses: the Cold Damage disorders (*shanghan*) tradition and the Warm Factor disorders (*wenbing*) tradition. Both continue to be practiced in contemporary Chinese medical clinics (Farquhar 1994: 107–31). In many regards Warm Factor doctrine is similar to that of the Cold Damage school, and the two traditions share such fundamental concepts of Chinese medicine as *yinyang*, *qi*, and the five phases (*wuxing*).[3] Although they have much in common, their explanations of the nature of exogenous heat illnesses are somewhat dissimilar, and this results in disparate methods of diagnosis and treatment.

Both doctrines follow classical principles in maintaining that the main cause of illness is an imbalance in the body's *qi*. *Qi* is a difficult concept to translate because it has a wide variety of associations and encompasses the functions, substances, and processes of the body. Perhaps the best way to understand *qi* is to use Nathan Sivin's straightforward language and then follow his example and leave the term untranslated. Sivin translates *qi* as the "basic stuff" of nature that both "makes things happen" and "in which things happen" (1987: 47). In the *Huangdi neijing* (Inner canon of the Yellow Lord), the foundational text of classical Chinese medicine, *qi* refers to both the materials and the processes of the human body that make vital functions possible.[4] It is also the force that causes illness (ibid.: 48–53). This dual quality of *qi* as the primary agent of both health and sickness is apparent in its conceptual division into orthopathic *qi* (*zheng qi*) and heteropathic *qi* (*xie qi*). Orthopathic *qi* encompasses "what is healthy and proper to the body," whereas heteropathic *qi* refers to "what is pathogenic and alien to it" (Kuriyama 1993: 54).

Good health continues as long as the body's orthopathic *qi* is robust, but an unequal distribution of orthopathic *qi* can be effected by a number of illness factors (*bingyin*). These include internal factors, such as excessive emotion (the seven emotional states, or *qi qing*); external factors brought on by seasonal change, atmospheric, or environmental conditions; and factors that are neither internal nor external, such as fatigue, improper diet, irregularity in personal hygiene, overindulgent alcohol consumption or sexual activity, and traumatic injury (Farquhar 1994: 88).[5]

While both the Cold Damage and Warm Factor schools adhere to these basic principles, they diverge in their explication of the nature and quality of the heteropathic *qi* thought to be responsible for the onset of exogenous heat illnesses. The Cold Damage scholarly line, which can be traced back to Zhang Ji's (Zhang Zhongjing, 196–220 C.E.) *Shanghan lun* (Treatise on Cold Damage disorders), incorporates the concepts of the six climatic configurations (*liu qi*) and the six excesses (*liu yin*) into its explanation of external illness factors. According to Cold Damage doctrine, the six climatic configurations (wind, cold, heat, moisture, dryness, and fire) cause no harm when they occur in proper sequence during seasonal cycles. In excess, or when they appear in the wrong season, they are transformed into the six excesses, and the resultant heteropathic *qi* can adversely affect those whose orthopathic *qi* is already weak (Sivin 1987: 275). Each of the six excesses is associated with a particular season according to the general philosophical principles of *yinyang* and the five phases (ibid.: 59–80).

Many Cold Damage disorders are, as the name implies, brought on by the heteropathic *qi* of excessive cold or wind. These climatic excesses are particularly dangerous because they can cause illness simultaneously among a large number of people within a particular area, as in an epidemic.[6] Even in such episodes, however, excessive cold and wind are not viewed as "disease agents" that act on all human anatomies in exactly the same way (Farquhar: 1994: 159–60). People may have similar symptoms, but diagnosis and treatment can never be separated from the particular condition of each patient's orthopathic *qi*.

The heteropathy enters the body through the pores of the skin and then works its way inward, killing the person when his or her heteropathic *qi* has sufficiently interfered with the body's vital functions. Practitioners of the Cold Damage doctrine divide this pathological process into six syndrome types (the six warps, or *liu jing*) according to the manifest symptoms, site of the illness, and its temporal stage. Six warps analysis thus allows for an evaluation of the seriousness of a patient's condition based on the location and progression of illness in the human body as well as the quality (cold) of the external illness factor involved. It is important to stress, however, that the spatial dimension is thought of in physiological rather than anatomical terms, and that the temporal sequence does not always follow a definite course (ibid.: 73).

Proponents of the Warm Factor tradition view the etiology and pathology of exogenous heat illnesses somewhat differently.[7] Drawing on the theories of Wu Youxing (Wu Youke, 1580's–1660's) as laid out in his 1642 *Wenyi lun* (Treatise on Warm Factor epidemics), Warm Factor practitioners do not believe that the six excesses (*liu yin*) are a factor in inducing illness at all.[8] Rather, they believe that the heteropathies which cause such illnesses are various kinds of pestilential *qi* (*li qi*) that can be present during any season and that enter the body through the mouth and nose as well as the pores of the skin. As a result many people in a discrete geographical area become sick, during episodes known as Warm Factor epidemics (*wenyi*).

Warm Factor practitioners employ a diagnostic technique known as "four sectors analysis" (*weiqi ying xue*). Developed in the eighteenth century, most prominently by Ye Gui (Ye Tianshi, 1667–1745) and Wu Tang (Wu Jutong, 1758–1836), four sectors diagnostics elucidate four pathological stages: the defensive sector (*wei*), the active sector (*qi*), the constructive sector (*ying*), and the blood sector (*xue*).[9] In addition, the technique incorporates the concept of the triple *jiao* (Triple Burners or *sanjiao*), using an ancient idea to describe upper, middle, and lower "cavities" in the body where Warm Factor disorders can stagnate. The three "cavities" are not seen as anatomical structures but are associated with particular bodily regions. The four sectors allow for temporal diagnosis according to the stage of development of the illness; the idea of three distinct regions of the body allows for therapeutics according to spatial position. Thus, as with the six warps diagnostics of the Cold Damage school, four sectors analysis allows for an evaluation of the severity of a patient's condition according to the location, direction (inward or outward, upward or downward), and speed of an illness process.

How the pestilential *qi* circulates and where it stagnates are the determining factors both in the development of any particular complex of symptoms and in the ultimate prognosis. The *qi* might, for example, coagulate in the superficial defensive sector (*wei*) of the upper cavity. The resulting complex of symptoms might include hot sensations, a stuffed and runny nose, coughing, and slight thirst—symptoms that biomedicine might identify as the common cold. At the other end of the spectrum, if the pestilential *qi* settles in the blood sector (*xue*) in the lower cavity, the disorder is very serious and the prognosis quite poor. Symptoms might include a very high fever, hemorrhaging, violent diarrhea and vomiting, purple or black spots on the skin, dementia, and convulsions. In biomedical nosography, these symptoms are often indicators of acute infectious diseases such as cholera or plague.

The Cold Damage and the Warm Factor traditions bring two distinct conceptual and diagnostic approaches to the same problem, namely, manifestations of exogenous heat illnesses. Although treating the same broad category of syndromes, the two schools describe the illness factor at work and the pathological processes in the human body quite differently. As a result, alternative treatment strategies are employed depending on the leanings of the particular physician. As Judith Farquhar (1994: 127–31) has demonstrated, in actual practice clinicians sometimes work out complex syntheses of the two. In scholarly discourse, however, there is much debate over the relative merits of each approach (ibid.: 130). Controversies and conflicts over the proper methods of syndrome differentiation and treatment determination of exogenous heat illnesses occurred frequently after the emergence of the Warm Factor tradition in the eighteenth century, and continue in academic medical circles today (Fang Yaozhong and Xu Jiasong 1986: 1).

Late-Qing Cold Damage and Warm Factor
Diagnoses of Plague

During the nineteenth- and early-twentieth-century plague epidemics in southeastern China, Chinese doctors, faced with a new and unfamiliar complex of symptoms, attempted to treat the disorder by using the diagnostic principles of either the Cold Damage or the Warm Factor lineage. Practitioners working in the Cold Damage tradition explained plague by looking for imbalances in the body's *qi*, seeking both deficiencies in orthopathic *qi* within the body and exogenous influences without. Diagnosis and treatment therefore consisted of careful and close monitoring of each patient and emphasis on personal hygiene, with less attention to the surrounding social environment. In contrast, Warm Factor physicians made connections between the polluted environment and widespread disease. In many ways this environmentalist approach resembled the miasmatic theory of infectious disease favored by European sanitarians in the mid-nineteenth century. In neither case, however, was contagion invoked as the cause of the disorder, as in the Western tradition.

The etiological thinking and diagnostic approach of Cold Damage practitioners with regard to plague are apparent in a late-Qing medical text entitled *Shuyi fei yi—liu jing tiaobian* (Plague is not an epidemic—Systematic manifestation type-determination in the Six Warps), written by Huang Zhongxian and published in 1909. Little is known about Huang Zhongxian except that he practiced medicine in Canton during the first decade of the twentieth century. Huang Zhongxian remained firmly committed to classical Cold Damage diagnostic methods in his treatment of plague. In his treatise he expressed dismay that, in writing about what was popularly termed *shuyi* (rat epidemic), so many medical texts emphasized only external heat factors and neglected the "proper" form of diagnosis through syndrome differentiation (*bianzheng*).

To treat the buboes (*hezheng*), Huang Zhongxian argued, physicians first had to be well schooled in classical Cold Damage theories and practice. It was essential to select the proper texts. He himself, he wrote, had examined the many published prescriptions that claimed to cure *shuyi* and had found that only those that treated Cold Damage were effective. As he put it, "Begin with this [Cold Damage] as the most important [principle] in order that the many people seeking medicine but who have not been properly diagnosed will increase their belief, those harmed will be without distress and will be cured, and will praise these prescriptions for their efficacy and power."

Huang Zhongxian was highly critical of Warm Factor practitioners, intimating that they were untrained, unprincipled quacks who offered only monocausal explanations of the illness factors underlying the syndrome and who did great harm through their misdiagnoses and inappropriate therapies. He argued that because the buboes appeared in many different forms (big or small, red or white, hard or soft) and in many disparate positions (high or low, in the *yin* or the *yang* tract) they could not possibly be induced by only one illness factor. In his opinion *shuyi* was emphatically not a Warm Factor epidemic (*wenyi*) caused by pestilential *qi* (*li qi*), but was caused by the heteropathic *qi* (*xie qi*) of the six excesses (*liu yin*). The bulk of Huang Zhongxian's treatise consists of a detailed explication of plague symptomatology using the six warps (*liu jing*) system of syndrome differentiation and treatment determination; the six sections of the text give appropriate prescriptions based on each of the six manifestations. His emphasis is on the careful and considered treatment of the individual patient, not the broader environmental context within which the person became ill.

Despite Huang Zhongxian's objections to it, the theory that plague was a Warm Factor epidemic appears to have won widespread acceptance in the late Qing, at least in southeastern China. During the late-nineteenth- and early-twentieth-century epidemics there, a Warm Factor treatise originally entitled *Zhi shuyi fa* (Methods for curing plague) was in extensive use throughout Fujian and Guangdong. Wu Zongxuan (Wu Xuecun), a scholar from Wuchuan county (Guangdong), wrote the first version in 1891 and presented it to Luo Rulan (Luo Zhi-yuan, from Shicheng county), who then edited the work, added his own prescriptions (*yaofang*) and case histories (*yi an*), and published it in 1895 under the title *Shuyi huibian* (Compilation on plague). Zheng Xiaoyan (1848–1920), a well-known physician from Minxian, Fujian, revised this second version still further, adding eight sections of prescriptions and medical cases and publishing the work in 1901 as *Shuyi yuebian* (A brief treatise on plague; Zheng Xiaoyan 1936 [1901]: preface).[10]

The section on illness factors in the *Shuyi yuebian*, originally crafted by Wu Zongxuan and later edited by Luo Rulan and Zheng Xiaoyan, provides an interpretation of plague based largely on the principles of the Warm Factor tradition of Chinese medicine (Zheng Xiaoyan 1936 [1901]: 1–3). The passage begins by criticizing those (i.e., Cold Damage practitioners) who still believed that plague was caused by the six climatic configurations (*liu qi*). Citing Wu Youxing (author of the *Wenyi lun*), the preface goes on to describe plague as a type of pestilential *qi* (*li qi*), in this case a visible, "turbid" *qi* (*zhuo qi*) that enters the body through the pores of the skin, the nose, or the mouth and that eventually stagnates in the blood sector (*xue*), thus cutting off the body's physical vitalities. The progression of symptoms in a particular patient indicates the point of entry of the pestilential *qi*, a factor that determines the patient's prognosis and that also suggests the proper course of treatment according to four sectors analysis. If buboes appear first and hot sensations develop only secondarily, then the *qi* has entered the body through the pores of the skin and is working its way, relatively slowly, from the defensive sector (*wei*) to the final blood sector (*xue*). If there are hot sensations first and then the buboes appear, the *qi* has entered the body through the nose or mouth and has attacked the blood sector almost immediately. Rapid deterioration follows, and death frequently occurs within three to five days.

The *Shuyi yuebian* further identifies the pestilential *qi* as an earthly (*di qi*) rather than an atmospheric *qi* (*tian qi*). This distinction provides an explanation for why rat epizootics occur before the outbreak of the disease among humans: Because the pestilential *qi* rises from the ground, it passes through rat burrows on its way to the surface. The rats are driven from their nests by the intense "heat" of the pestilential *qi*. Seeking relief, the animals drink from water cisterns or even unattended teacups. When humans unwittingly drink from the same containers, they receive the pestilential *qi*.

Based on their observation that the disease had its origins in an earthly, "turbid" *qi*, Wu Zongxuan, Luo Rulan, and Zheng Xiaoyan advocated improvements in household sanitation as well as personal hygiene. According to the *Shuyi yuebian*, preventive measures are necessary because once the epidemic begins there is "no way to treat it." The best prevention is to clean the house and be on guard against rats. The windows must be kept open to allow cleansing breezes to sweep away any pestilential *qi*. Dark and damp places are to be avoided, as is yellow or stagnant water. Any dead rats must be buried immediately, while keeping the nose carefully covered. People are not to sit on the floor or on beds that touch the floor for fear that the earthly *qi* will infect them. Shoes are recommended to keep the feet away from direct contact with the *qi*, and limits are advised on the number of people allowed to crowd into one room.

The treatise also advocates that, as a preventive measure, people leave urban areas and go to the countryside to get away from the unhealthy air of the cities. Wealthy people who shut themselves up during epidemics are urged to open their windows and doors to let the wind in. To underscore the therapeutic benefits of improved ventilation, the *Shuyi yuebian* notes that, although many people contract plague when they go to market, those who open the flaps on their sedan chairs are likely to recover completely, while those who keep their chairs tightly closed almost certainly die. The treatise then relates the story of a man, taken for dead, who was about to be closed up in his coffin. Fortunately for him, a thief stole his burial clothes in the night and the cooling breezes he received allowed him to recover completely.

In their interpretations of plague and the preventive measures they advocated, Warm Factor physicians had a great deal in common with some of their nineteenth-century Western counterparts. In the 1890's, the etiology of plague was only beginning to be understood by Western scientists. Until about 1880, many researchers favored environmentalist theories of communicable diseases such as plague, retaining and elaborating on the belief that miasmas arising from stagnant water and odorous sewage engendered epidemics (Ackerknecht 1948: 562–93; Duffy 1993: 202–4). The miasmatic view of infectious disease was the basis for many of the sanitary reforms carried out in Europe and North America in the mid-nineteenth century (see Chapter 5). Although the triumph of the germ theory in the last quarter of the nineteenth century led to the identification in 1894 of the specific bacterial agent that causes plague, controversy remained over its precise mode of transmission and the most effective means of combatting it (Hirst 1953:

106–20). Many practicing physicians and laypeople continued to believe that plague was a miasmal "filth" disease caused by inadequate ventilation and poor drainage. Western physicians advocated environmental and household cleaning, better waterworks, sewage treatment, and fresh air as the principal means of combatting the epidemic. Only after it was shown that bubonic plague is transmitted to humans by rat fleas did prevention efforts focus on exterminating and controlling the actual vectors.

The emphasis of the Warm Factor doctors on improved ventilation and housecleaning suggests that they may have been influenced by Western ideas. Indeed, the *Shuyi yuebian* urges its readers to follow the "foreign" method of periodically cooling off beneath a tree or on a lake. Luo Rulan even suggests that the "new" method of isolating plague patients be tried in China, although he does not say why he believes this might be efficacious. While the Warm Factor writings on plague may have borrowed from contemporary European thinking on the subject, foreign ideas were also adapted to fit the basic principles of the Warm Factor tradition. Where both the Cold Damage and the Warm Factor medical doctrines differed from European conceptions of disease was in the area of contagion. Despite Luo Rulan's tentative suggestion that quarantine be implemented, neither tradition located the source of the illness in the body of the patient, so neither seriously advocated either restrictions on movement or the removal of plague patients from their families.

I have drawn a strict dichotomy between the Cold Damage and Warm Factor traditions to underscore the complexity of late-nineteenth-century Chinese medical ideas about the nature of plague. Some physicians, such as Huang Zhongxian, adhered strictly to the diagnostic and treatment methods of one or the other doctrine because they believed such techniques were highly effective. But most doctors no doubt borrowed from both, relying on their own practical experience (and that of their predecessors, as transmitted in texts) to determine the appropriate approach in particular cases (Farquhar 1994: 131). The wranglings between Cold Damage and Warm Factor practitioners were of little concern to most Chinese patients, who probably chose their doctors on the basis of their reputations rather than their theoretical orientations and clinical procedures. More to the point, distinctions between Cold Damage and Warm Factor doctors were largely irrelevant for the peasant majority, who had no access to elite medical care. For many if not most Chinese living in the nineteenth century, the plague epidemics were supernatural phenomena requiring the intervention of spirit mediums, Daoist priests, Buddhist clerics, or other ritual specialists.

Popular Beliefs About the Origins of Plague

Popular beliefs about the etiology of plague were rooted both in an ancient tradition that linked disease to dangerous external forces and in a more recent tradition that viewed epidemics as a form of divine retribution for immoral behavior. The first identifiably Chinese conception of epidemic disease, developed during the Shang dynasty (sixteenth-eleventh centuries B.C.E.) and refined during the early Zhou (ca. 1066–771), concentrated on ancestral spirits or demons that threatened the body from without (Kuriyama 1993: 52; Unschuld 1985: 17–50). The earliest Chinese therapeutics consisted of exorcistic rituals, magical incantations, and the preparation of lucky talismans designed to purge the body of these spirits. Although new conceptions of disease arose as China entered the imperial age, ancestral and demonological medicine continued as important "thematic poles to which reflections on sickness would repeatedly return" (Kuriyama 1993: 52).

The belief that epidemics served as divine punishment for the moral failings of individual people emerged in the late Han (25–220 C.E.) and the Six Dynasties (222–589) periods, when popular forms of religious Daoism and Buddhism began to be widely accepted among commoners (Kuriyama 1993: 56). By the twelfth century this belief was well established in much of China. Gradually, popular religious ideas emerged that linked Confucian values with the idea of divine intervention. Adherents conceptualized a heavenly bureaucracy within which there was a Ministry of Epidemics (*Wenbu*) presided over by five deities known as the Five Commissioners of Epidemics (*Wuwen shizhe*; see Katz 1987: 207–8 and 1990: 98–106). Good health was viewed as the gods' reward for meritorious acts, and illness as retaliation for bad ones. These celestial bureaucrats kept track of each person's merits and demerits, and when transgressions became too great, disease was sent as punishment. Epidemics occurred when the divine bureaucracy deemed an entire community to be beyond redemption.

These two interpretations of disease informed common understanding of the nineteenth-century plague epidemics. In the popular imagination, plague was both the work of uncontrollable "epidemic demons" (*yigui*) and an affliction imposed on "evil" communities by powerful "plague gods" (*wenshen*) acting as emissaries of the Five

Commissioners of Epidemics.[11] As with other supernatural beings in the Chinese pantheon, *yigui* and *wenshen* were believed to be in a hierarchical relationship. *Yigui*, at the very bottom of the hierarchy, were conceived of as the vengeful, wandering spirits of people who had died premature or violent deaths. Like other "hungry ghosts" (*ligui*), *yigui* roamed the countryside, seeking comfort from the living. The early-Qing statecraft writer Yuan Yixiang described epidemic ghosts as follows:[12]

There are those who died in water, fire, or were killed by robbers . . . those who have had their property taken away and who have committed suicide as a result. There are those whose wives have been forcibly taken away by others and who have then died. There are criminals who have died in shame, those who have starved or frozen to death. These are all ghosts whose souls have not dispersed. Their spirits are silent and lonely and cannot return home. They are left in suspension, hoping for rites. (He Changling 1886, 45: 2a–3b)

When the human population ignored them and did not offer the proper ritual sacrifices, these ghosts spread miasmal vapors designed to kill the population in epidemics. Ironically, those who died in epidemics also became wandering ghosts capable of creating disastrous epidemics in turn ([*Xuxiu*] *Menghua zhiliting zhi* 1790, 2: 99).

There were innumerable stories about the ghosts that brought epidemic disease, and each locality no doubt had its own (Katz 1990: 108). Two examples will perhaps give a sense of the variety of these tales. An account from a Guangxi gazetteer tells about the ghostly origins of epidemic disease in Baishan township:

In 1756 [Qianlong 21], a peasant named Old Deng and several of his companions were at a pond getting water when suddenly they saw a human figure that was about two feet [two *chi*] tall, riding on a beast that looked like a sheep and leading about ten other beings who were the same size. When they arrived at the pond, they said to Old Deng, "We are going to the capital of Baishansi." Then they headed off in the direction of the town. Old Deng and his companions were fearful, but they followed behind anyway in order to spy on them. Suddenly, the *yin* wind rose on all sides and the creatures disappeared. Not many days later, the capital of Baishansi suffered an epidemic. (*Baishansi zhi* 1830, 16: 5a–5b)

Another story comes from Yunnan and provides an explanation for the mid-nineteenth-century plague epidemics there:

Just before the epidemic spread [through Yunnan], the people all saw a ghostly fire of several thousand ghosts marching in military formation through the night. When the ghosts approached closer, the people could hear the sound of gongs, drums, bells, horns, horses' hoofs, and the sound of weapons clanging. The apparition of flags and pennants could be seen in the moonlight. As the ghosts came closer, people fell to the ground as if they were in a trance. The next day, after they revived, they said that they had been conscripted by the ghosts to carry their goods. . . . After several days . . . the epidemic began. (Yu Yue 1935, 2: 130).

These two stories reveal the attributes of the epidemic ghosts that made them so dangerous. They roamed in packs: Old Deng and his companions saw eleven ghosts, and villagers in Yunnan saw thousands of them. Unlike an ordinary illness, which might be caused by one hungry ghost, epidemic disease was brought by a multitude of them, and hence many people became ill at the same time. In the tale from Guangxi, seemingly innocuous creatures (only two feet high) turn out to be very dangerous. In the story from Yunnan, the ghosts were represented as malevolent spirit-soldiers who marched on the village bringing disease, very much no doubt, in the manner in which the rat-infested baggage of real soldiers brought plague to the villages in Yunnan.

Yigui could act on their own, but they more commonly served as functionaries for the more powerful epidemic gods (*wenshen*). There was no one "God of Plague"; rather, many different cults of *wenshen* spread throughout southern China. Liu Zhiwan (1962: 715) has described *wenshen* rituals as they are practiced in contemporary Taiwan and has shown that *wenshen* temples were common in Fujian, Guangdong, Hunan, and Jiangsu.[13] Paul Katz (1990; 1991) has documented the rituals associated with one such plague deity, Marshall Wen (Wen Yuanshuai), who was widely worshiped in Zhejiang. Local gazetteers of Guangxi, Guizhou, and Yunnan show that rituals and practices similar to those described by Liu Zhiwan and Katz for southeastern China existed historically in the southwest as well. This is not surprising because Han immigrants no doubt carried images of *wenshen* with them as they moved from the southeast into Guizhou and Yunnan.[14] During the 1811 plague epidemic in Shiping county in Yunnan, for example, residents worshiped the image of a plague god they had brought from Hubei (*Shipingxian zhi* 1938: 18b–19b).

Many people, particularly practicing Buddhists and religious Daoists, believed that the gods sent plague as a punishment for moral depravity (Katz 1990: 171). This was the message of the planchette (*fuji*) revelations of Huang Daxian (Wong Tai Sin), a god whose cult originated in Canton in the 1890's largely as a result of the plague epidemics there (Lang and Ragvald 1993: 13–15). According to this god's messages, plague was due to evil deeds:

[The plague], which produces such a horrifying scene [of crowds of people desperately beseeching the god] is actually caused by the wrong-doing of the people. It is due to their misbehaviour that Heaven sends this kind of epidemic disease to fill up this whole region. . . . Nowadays, . . . [even] among brothers there is suspicion and murder. Indecent sexual behaviour, theft, lies, and fraud are common. These acts bring people nearer to death. How can people pursue immorality? (ibid.: 15–16; brackets in original translation)

A similar description of the origins of the plague appeared in a proclamation said to have been received through the planchette from Guandi (Guan Yu), the God of War (Ball 1895; Unschuld 1985: 226–28).[15] The planchette revelations were circulated in 1894 by a Cantonese charitable organization. Guandi stated through the planchette that, in order to forewarn the righteous, he had chosen to divulge heaven's design to annihilate the sinful:

Heaven was exasperated and said that the world was overcrowded with people and had been for a long time increasingly harbouring wicked men; that even a small child of three feet in height was also full of evil deeds. Heaven had ordered . . . floods in the rivers, winds, waters, fire, and pestilence, which were to scourge and destroy more than one half of the population. (Ball 1895: 236)

Guandi's revelations indicated that he had taken pity on humanity and had intervened enough to reduce the punishment to a half year of pestilence only. The planchette also revealed that Guandi had been made the "Assistant Superintendent" of the "Ministry Governing Epidemics" (*Wenbu*) and that he had been placed in charge of a hundred inspectors of merits and demerits, a thousand plague gods, and innumerable plague demons who were to go among the people to examine their deeds and mete out punishments. The plague would only cease when five thousand families in each city or town had repented and demonstrated evidence of good deeds. The wealthy were to subscribe to benevolent associations and the poor to recite the proper liturgies to show their sincerity.

While Guandi's planchette revelations were informed largely by Buddhist values, Confucian ideals were included as well. Guandi promised that the plague would not harm those who were filial to their parents and true to their friends. Nor were practical remedies overlooked: the planchette provided information on how to safely lance the buboes, and it included a prescription guaranteed to be efficacious in

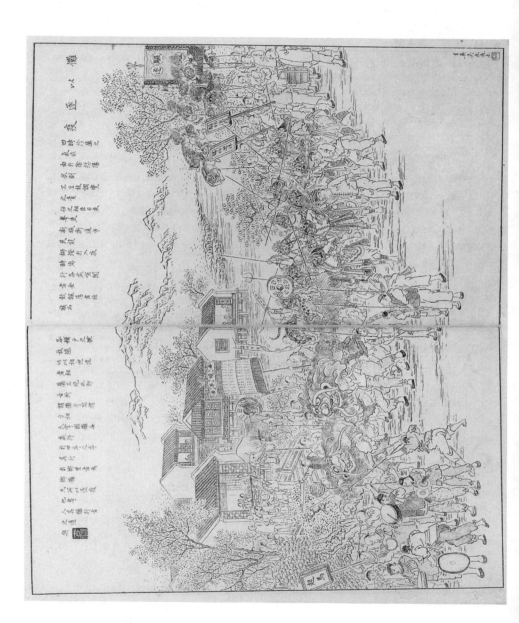

treatment of the disease. Guandi also advised that well water be puri-fied with garlic and insecticidal drugs because it had become polluted by the "filth" of dead rats. Guandi closed the planchette by promis-ing to personally treat those who were truly sincere and faithful. As Paul Unschuld (1985: 228) has pointed out, this document reveals that the wide diversity of Chinese conceptions of disease (medical and religious, natural and supernatural) could easily be believed simulta-neously and without contradiction. It also suggests the ways in which these varied etiological beliefs gave rise to multiple responses within plague-infected communities.

Community Responses to Plague

Given the centrality of gods and demons in popular thinking about epidemics, collective efforts at plague eradication centered on exor-cistic *jiao* (offering rites) aimed at placating the *wenshen* and driving away the *yigui*.[16] Ritual plague-god festivals (*wenshen jiao*) were peri-odically held in many communities as prophylactic measures against epidemics; similar rituals were held after an epidemic had broken out. Lasting about a week, the *jiao* included days of elaborate temple rites and liturgies, culminating in a large processional designed to expel all remaining plague demons and send the plague god back to heaven (Figure 8). This was done by placing the *wenshen* on mas-sive boats (*wenchuan*) made of paper or grass that were then burnt or floated away.[17]

The custom of burning an effigy of plague gods on boats appears to have originated in southeastern China and was most widespread in Fujian, Taiwan, and Zhejiang, but the burning of plague gods was conducted in other parts of southern China as well.[18] In Yunnan and Guizhou antiepidemic *Qing jiao* ("cleansing rituals") were celebrated on the second day of the third month, the birthday of Wen Chang. While *Qing jiao* were used elsewhere for the more generalized function of protecting the community from all disasters, the explicitly stated purpose of these *jiao* was the prevention of epidemics. In this the *Qing jiao* of the southwest resemble the *Wang jiao* of Taiwan and Fujian,

---

FIG. 8 (*opposite*). "A festival to drive out the epidemic." Nineteenth-century woodcut depicting a plague god festival (*wenshen jiao*) in Xincheng, a town in the eastern part of Guangdong. From *Dianshizhai huabao* 1983 [1885] 4/*ding*.9: 70. Courtesy of the Library of Congress.

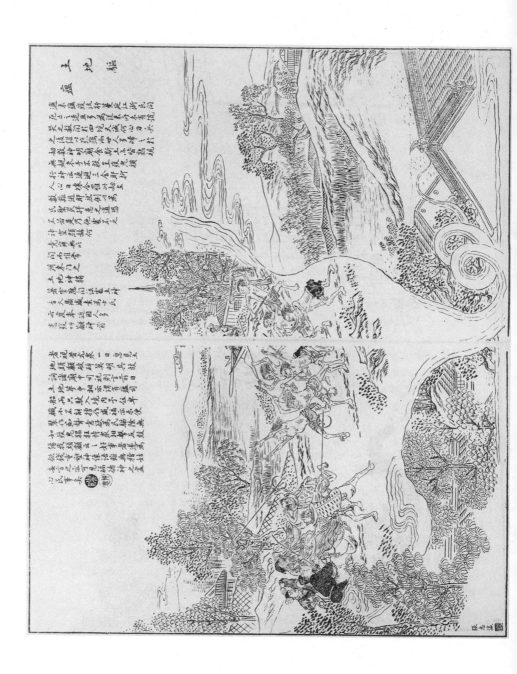

which were celebrated in the fourth lunar month, and the Marshall Wen *jiao* of Zhejiang, which were celebrated during the third lunar month (Katz 1991; Liu Zhiwan 1983). A description of the *Qing jiao* in Guizhou reads:[19]

Every spring, in the towns and countryside, people pool their money in order to hold a *Qing jiao*. They use paper to make a dragon boat, spirit mediums use red ink to paint their faces like each god in the pantheon. They seek out the fugitives [ghosts] at each household along the way in order to exorcise epidemics. (*Bijiexian zhi* 1879, 7: 9a)

In each locality, particular gods were reputed to have the power to halt epidemics. The text accompanying Figure 9 describes a fight between the local god of Dongmen county (in Changzhou prefecture, Jiangsu) and epidemic ghosts who had arrived on two plague boats. Even this "uniquely powerful" god was unable to vanquish the ghosts, who were so fierce that they damaged the head of his statue. When local gods failed to lift the plague, as in this instance, one response was to bring in more powerful gods from elsewhere (Figure 10). In 1894 Zhou Sicheng, a man from Mengzi, traveled to Jiangxi to bring back the image of Kang Da Yuanshuai, an action that was reputedly the reason the plague finally stopped there ([*Xu*] *Mengzixian zhi* 1961 [1911], 12: 43b). Cantonese community leaders, believing that an image of Bao Gong enshrined at a temple in Zhaoqing prefecture would drive away plague demons, petitioned the magistrate to allow this image to be transported to Canton. He consented, money was collected for the expenses of the god's trip, and it was paraded through the streets of the city (*North China Herald* [hereafter *NCH*], June 15, 1894: 946).[20] When plague appeared in Xiangshan county in 1898, local leaders also brought in a god from elsewhere and set up a new temple in his honor (*Xiangshanxian zhi* 1923, 16: 7). Another common strategy was to declare a new year, thereby tricking the plague gods into thinking that the time for bringing pestilence had not yet arrived (Goodrich 1964:

FIG. 9 (*opposite*). "The local god dispels the epidemic." This woodcut relates the story of a battle between epidemic ghosts and the local god of Dongmen county (in Changzhou prefecture, Jiangsu). The text explains that the god felt compelled to drive out the epidemic ghosts even though "his own position was so low that he could not punish or reward according to his own whim." As a result of the brawl, the head of the god's statue in the local temple was broken, necessitating repairs financed by local philanthropists. From *Dianshizhai huabao* 1983 [1895] 36/*shu*.2: 13. Courtesy of the Library of Congress.

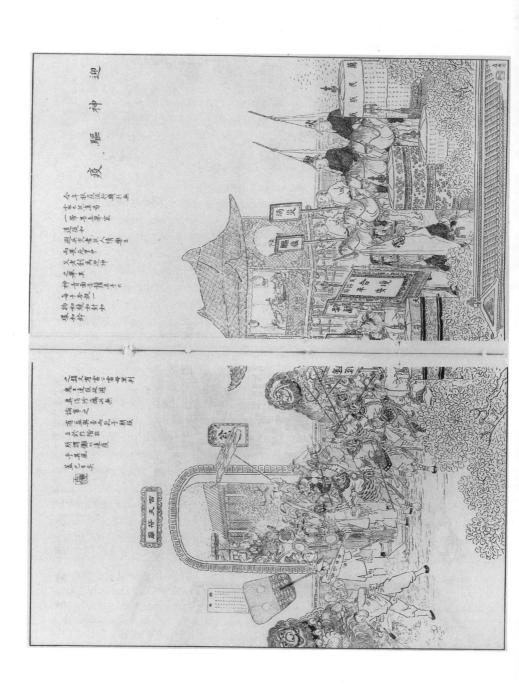

116; Katz 1987: 209). This practice was followed in Lingui county in Guangxi as well as in Canton in 1894 (Inspectorate General, *Customs Medical Reports* 1894, No. 48: 71–72; *Linguixian zhi* 1905, 18: 282).

For the most part, religious festivals provided spiritual comfort but did little to prevent or slow the spread of epidemics. Indeed, during epidemics of communicable disease, the large congregations that gathered at ritual ceremonies may have exacerbated the rate of infection by carrying disease back to their local communities.[21] Along with religious rituals, however, there were customary communal practices that had the practical effect of protecting the public's health. In Yunnan, local communities reportedly stationed guards along major trade routes to prevent travelers from passing during epidemics or the malaria season (Cooper 1871a: 165). A French priest who had lived in Yunnan for "many years" confirmed that, prior to the Muslim Rebellion (which had "destroyed every organization" in the province), it had been customary for towns to post guards on the road to prevent anyone from entering "during the unhealthy season" (Gill 1883: 274). In some communities, local leaders had stone walls built within a town to isolate infected neighborhoods from those not yet infected (*Linguixian zhi* 1905, 18: 282).[22]

The five deities who were said to preside over the Ministry of Epidemics (*Wenbu*) were thought to make their inspection tour of Earth during the first five days of the fifth lunar month, and thus Duanwu (the Dragon Boat Festival) was a day when households undertook precautions against the epidemic diseases expected in the summer months ahead. In contemporary China, the Dragon Boat Festival is viewed as a commemoration of Qu Yuan's loyalty (lived ca. 340–290 B.C.E.), but the boat races themselves, now the centerpiece of any celebration of Duanwu, probably had their origin in exorcistic rituals designed to rid a community of epidemic spirits (Chao 1943; Katz 1987: 209). People also warded off demons on Duanwu by drinking wine made from realgar, orpiment (arsenic trisulphide), Acorus calamas, or mugwort (artemisia vulgaris). These chemicals were also sprinkled around the house because residents believed they killed insects and snakes.[23]

When epidemic disease did break out, individual households immediately took steps to protect themselves. One strategy was to post

---

FIG. 10 (*opposite*). "Welcoming the god to dispel the epidemic." Woodcut depicting the arrival of a new god and the processional of his statue. From *Dianshizhai huabao* 1983 [1885] 5/*wu*.6: 42. Courtesy of the Library of Congress.

couplets on their front gateways (even if no one was sick) in an attempt to trick the plague gods or demons into believing that the household had already been afflicted or to persuade them to move on. The couplets generally consisted of phrases such as "The heavenly travelers have passed" (*Tian xing yi guo*), meaning that another deity had already deemed the house righteous enough to be passed over (Katz 1990: 241). The 1894 planchette revelations of Guandi, for example, suggested that his followers should paste on their doors a couplet with the words "Assistant Superintendent of the Ministry Governing Epidemics" along with his seal. This, the planchette promised, would prevent the plague demons from entering (Ball 1895: 235). In Guangxi, this practice seemed also to serve as a kind of voluntary quarantine. Several Guangxi gazetteers note that it was customary to post notices outside the gate to alert visitors that a person inside was ill (*Hechizhou zhi* 1907, *fengsu* [customs]: 1a; *Qingyuanfu zhi* 1829, 3: 1b). Of course, this might also have been a ploy by a healthy household to prevent infected persons from entering.

Certain practices were inspired by religious beliefs but had practical public-health consequences. For example, people swept out their houses and streets to make the neighborhood more hospitable to gods who had the power of lifting the epidemic, or to illustrate their contrition for past sins (Hsu 1952: 46–47; Katz 1990: 186). Similarly, to welcome supernatural entities, families sought to keep public water supplies clean by voluntarily refraining from washing food or clothes in them. As Paul Katz (1990: 77–79) has pointed out, the cleanliness of wells was always a central concern during epidemics, and rumors of well-poisonings were common. Plague demons were often identified as the culprits, but "outsiders" were accused of well-poisoning just as frequently. Foreign missionaries in particular were held suspect in this regard (*Liujiangxian zhi* 1937: 199).

In their search for pure water, people flocked to the many mountain springs reputed to have miraculous healing qualities: a spring in the eastern part of Mengzi county in Yunnan was believed to cure plague ([*Xu*] *Mengzixian zhi* 1961 [1911], 12: 36a; see also accounts of healing waters in *Dalixian zhigao* 1917, 24: 27a; *Pu'erfu zhi* 1850 [1840], 20: 4a). Sometimes the miraculous water was carted into the city and sold (Hsu 1952: 51–55). Families also sought to purify their own houses by burning realgar or arsenic trisulfide inside the house. The sulfuric smoke these chemicals produced was thought to be effective in removing pestilential *qi* (Rocher 1879, 2: 280; [*Xu*] *Mengzixian zhi* 1961

[1911], 12: 43b; [*Xuxiu*] *Jianshuixian zhigao* 1920, 10: 22a). Another tradition that seems to have a long history was boiling or burning the clothes of those who died during epidemics.[24]

After an outbreak of disease, handwritten or printed notices appeared (often prepared by religious organizations) offering medical and moral advice on how to avoid the epidemic. People were urged to copy down the contents of the notices and pass them around, an act that counted as a "good deed" for which they would receive heavenly merit. In the planchette mentioned earlier, Guandi instructed his followers to distribute twenty copies of his revelations in order to save themselves, and two hundred copies to save their entire families (Ball 1895: 236). One common admonition in these circulars was that people abstain from meat-eating and sexual activity. Rocher (1879, 2: 280) noted that this was a common response in Yunnan between 1871 and 1873, and in 1891 placards were posted all over Mengzi after an epidemic broke out, prohibiting the butchering of cattle for food (Inspectorate General, *Decennial Reports* 1882–91: 671). Benevolent institutions also printed and distributed broadsheets listing medical prescriptions thought to be effective in curing plague. The *Shuyi yuebian*, the late-nineteenth-century treatise on plague already discussed, was widely circulated throughout the southeast in this manner, and a temple committee in Hong Kong distributed ten thousand copies of another circular that originated in Yunnan and that included the prescriptions of a Chinese doctor "who allegedly had cured a number of plague victims" (Sinn 1989: 162).

Despite the claims of wonder drugs that were said to cure plague, the disease exacted a heavy toll in many of the communities it afflicted. As the number of deaths increased, reactions became more desperate. Some residents began to place the dead or dying out on the street (Inspectorate General, *Customs Medical Reports* 1894, No. 48: 46). During such a crisis there was little time to perform the proper funerary rites, such as ceremonially sealing the corpses in airtight coffins (*Dataoxian zhi* 1845, 2: 58b). Abandonment of the dead and dying along the sides of the roads was all too common during epidemics, and testifies to the terror such a crisis must have engendered in a community. In the most extreme instances, entire communities fled, leaving their villages or towns deserted.[25]

Official Responses to Plague

Although the eighteenth-century Qing state maintained an elaborate and extensive famine-relief system (Will 1990; Will and Wong 1991), aid during epidemics was generally considered a routine task best handled by the local district magistrate. Unlike famines and floods, which typically affected broad stretches of territory, epidemics rarely occurred over a wide enough area to be considered truly catastrophic. Moreover, because disease was always present to some extent, it was probably not easy for officials to recognize when an epidemic was first underway. The localized nature of epidemics, combined with the difficulties and subjectivities inherent in distinguishing "abnormal" levels of sickness, meant that epidemics seldom warranted much attention in memorials sent to Beijing. In contrast to the extensive Qing reportage on famines caused by flood or drought (Will 1990: 7–17), extant memorials regarding epidemics are very rare.[26]

Official neglect appears to have extended even to reportage of the widespread outbreaks of plague in the eighteenth and nineteenth centuries. Extensive research in the Number One Historical Archives in Beijing turned up only a handful of memorials related to epidemic relief efforts, and only one of these, an 1814 memorial written by Yunnan Provincial Educational Commissioner Gu Chun, is clearly related to plague (*Gongzhongdang, Zhupi zuozhe, Wenjiaolei, yiyao weisheng* [hereafter *GZD I*], Gu Chun, Jiaqing 19/9/6 [1814] group 4, doc. 207–23; see Chapter 1). In this memorial, Gu Chun describes how he distributed special medicine to plague victims in Lin'an prefecture after conducting a thorough investigation of the epidemic in the area.

Based on the few reports that do exist of official activities during epidemics, it is clear that Gu Chun's response was a typical one. The standard Qing administrative practice during epidemics was to conduct an investigation and then distribute medicine free of charge (Leung 1987: 141–42). This two-stage policy of investigation and relief was clearly modeled on long-standing famine prevention programs (Will 1990). As in the case of drought or flood, the local magistrate was supposed to report an epidemic to his superiors without delay. An imperial endorsement to a memorial reporting an epidemic in Anhui province in 1821 (in all likelihood of cholera) expresses the imperial expectations for such expediency:

Whenever epidemics occur in localities, then officials should memorialize. We have heard of some officials who wait two months to report, or who sit on the required notification for a long time. Doctors in the capital have efficacious remedies [so] let [this] be known. We already know that the epidemics are thick in the south and that many die. There are those who are shirking their duty. Henceforth, officials must devote their entire energy to [relieving] the people's suffering, and manage [relief] according to the situation. Those who have not carried out their duty must not fail again. (*GZD I*, Vermilion endorsement to Zhang Shicheng enclosure, Daoguang 1/9/3 [1821], group 4, doc. 207.26)

After the investigation, officials were required to post yellow notices (*tenghuang*) displaying any imperial commands and any intended relief efforts.[27] Failure to post such notices was also cause for punishment, and a delay of more than a month meant dismissal from office (Metzger 1973: 163). Local officials had the prerogative of exempting any area stricken by epidemic disease from tax payments.[28]

Following an investigation, local officials donated medicine to those affected by the epidemic, either directly through the magistrate's office or through semiofficial charitable dispensaries (*shiyao ju*).[29] One such dispensary in Kunming collected and distributed donations of money and medicine during the 1870's epidemics there.[30] In addition, the dispensary printed and distributed handbills describing prescriptions thought to be efficacious in treating the disease (*Kunmingxian zhi* 1939, 2: 13a–14b). Officials, acting in the manner of local gentry, also made personal contributions of money, food, and medicine directly to victims, and they solicited contributions from wealthy elite to help defray the costs of public charity.[31]

There is some indication that a network existed for the long-distance transport of medicine, at least for soldiers and officials serving in remote locations. Local officials were required to report any particularly effective remedy discovered in their districts to the central Taiyiyuan (Imperial Medical Bureau; see Gong Chun 1959; 1960).[32] They were also required to send such medicines in bulk to the capital for storage. For the most part, the drugs sent to the capital were used by members of the Imperial Household. In some cases, however, this medicine was redirected to places that needed it to treat victims during epidemics. If the medicine required was not available locally, provincial officials memorialized Beijing for extra supplies.[33]

In 1769 the Grand Council (*Junji chu*) attempted to deal with the problem of disease (probably malaria) among officials serving in Yunnan by commissioning the governor-general of Guangxi and Guangdong, Li Shiyao, to procure medicine from foreign merchants in Canton. Li Shiyao was instructed to buy the highest quality *awei* from the foreigners and send it to Mingde, the governor of Yunnan (Yunnan-sheng lishi yanjiusuo 1984, 4: 729).[34] Li Shiyao went to the foreign merchants and asked about their method of production of the drug and its use. He was told that *awei* came from the sap of a tree which, when congealed and used as a plaster on the chest, could prevent disease. Li Shiyao proceeded to buy 3,000 *jin* (approximately 3,000 pounds) of *awei* and shipped it, as instructed, to Yunnan (*GZD I*, Li Shiyao memorial, Qianlong 34/2/7 [1769], group 4, doc. 207.10). Mingde was properly appreciative, memorializing that:

> I have investigated the drug *awei* and have found that it can prevent *zhangqi* [miasmas]. Along the border, the people of that region all know about [this drug]. But it is not produced in Yunnan and it is unusual for foreign merchants to come here. These past two or three years, it has been completely sold out. Not only do local officials and soldiers have difficulty buying it, even I myself surprisingly cannot buy it. Now due to the fact our emperor loves and pities his people he has directed the governor-general of Lingnan, Li Shiyao, to send three thousand *jin* of *awei* to Yunnan. I have ordered that the *awei* be taken to those places that need it. (*GZD I*, Mingde memorial, Qianlong 34/5/23 [1769], group 4, doc. 207.11).

Such official concern was intended not only to protect the health of officials and soldiers in the border regions but also to ensure that social order was maintained. In a later memorial Mingde noted:

> The three thousand *jin* of *awei* sent from Guangdong to Tengyue has been distributed. [I] have investigated the border areas. Although there is *zhangqi* there, there are also many rumors about it. People have become suspicious and afraid. Now that we have allowed the people to obtain effective medicine to avoid the *zhangqi*, not only have we protected their health, but we have alleviated suspicion and fear. This is a great help to the military officials. (Yunnansheng lishi yanjiusuo 1984, 4: 729)

Concerns over possible threats to social order during epidemics prompted the particular attention paid to prisoners during such episodes. The local jail was highly susceptible to outbreaks of infectious disease. Magistrates' handbooks described how prisoners should be treated in the event of outbreaks of epidemics (Xu Wenbi 1976 [Qing], 1: n.p.). In 1818 a Yunnanese official, Bo Lin, memorialized the Grand Secretariat (*Neige*), reporting that an epidemic (possibly of plague) was spreading through the area around Jianshui. He reported that many prisoners had already died and that he had accordingly reduced the number of prison guards by half. He also threatened to impeach any prison warden who maltreated prisoners by denying them medical attention or food (Yunnansheng lishi yanjiusuo 1984, 4: 565). Sometimes prisoners were released and allowed to return home during epidemics.

In addition to providing medical charity, officials ordered that certain measures beneficial to the public's health be carried out. Common provisos included sweeping and repairing public thoroughfares, dredging the communal well, and burning the personal effects of plague victims.[35] Bo Lin ordered laborers to sweep the streets of Jianshui after the 1818 outbreak (Yunnansheng lishi yanjiusuo 1984, 4: 565). Magistrates also ordered that the corpses of plague victims be buried as quickly as possible.[36] Officials were motivated in large part by the belief that unburied corpses were the source of heteropathic *qi*.[37] Huang Liuhong (Huang Liu-hung), in his seventeenth-century handbook for local magistrates, outlines the proper way to conduct burials during an epidemic:

> On occasions when plagues [epidemics] strike, many victims die; their corpses fill the roads and ditches and give out a terrible stench. It is the magistrate's duty to provide burial land for these unfortunate souls. He should purchase land, preferably from his own allowance or by soliciting voluntary contributions from wealthy families, to provide free cemeteries. Coffins of poor people and travelers without claimants are permitted to be buried there. Unburied coffins with no claimants or identification found in the wilderness or in temples should be reported by the village headman or the monks of the temples and immediately buried in the free cemetery.
>
> When a number of people die in a plague, surviving relatives of the victims will bury their dead, but victims without surviving relatives will have to be buried by the government. If there are enough contributions from philanthropists, these victims will be buried in coffins. If not, the village headmen or the monks will have to bury them in deep pits. A wooden sign describing the deceased's age, appearance, and clothing should mark the grave. The number of burials should be reported to the magistrate's yamen. If the corpses are buried in shallow pits, dogs or wild animals may dig them up and leave the bones exposed, and the village headman or the monks who conducted the burial should be held responsible. A kind-hearted magistrate will not feel comfortable when there are exposed bones within his jurisdiction. (Huang Liu-hung 1984: 554)

The fact that magistrates took this responsibility seriously is underscored by the fact that memorialists often reported that they had provided for charitable burials in their districts (*Gongzhongdang, Zhupi zouzhe, Neizheng lei, zhenji* [hereafter *GZD II*], Qing Bao memorial, Jiaqing 19/3/30 [1814], group 359-4-75, box 78).

Proper worship of the plague gods, it was believed, could also prevent epidemics from breaking out, and local magistrates were expected to conduct the rituals that would guarantee the future safety of the community. Regular offerings were made to the City God (*Chenghuang shen*) at the Altar for Vengeful Souls (*Litan*), situated in the northern part of each administrative unit (Katz 1991: 24). The City God was appealed to during other natural disasters as well, but neglect of this deity could bring on the wrath of "vengeful souls" in the form of pestilence. In 1660 Yuan Yixiang chided local officials in Shaoxing prefecture (in Zhejiang) for their neglect of the rituals that would appease the City God:

> The lonely ghosts are left suspended, hoping for rites. There are temples that provide them sanctuary; the principal one is that of the City God. Now, although these exist in name, there are some temples that do not make offerings to the lonely ghosts. The ghosts will vent their resentment and become manifest as epidemics . . . this [worship] is beyond the worship of the God of Crops. . . . From this time on, every year during Qing-Ming festival, during the mid-Autumn festival, and in the tenth month of the year, it is necessary for officials to personally worship [the lonely ghosts]. The lonely ghosts will then be at peace and will not create disaster. (He Changling 1886, 45: 2b)

Officials also joined with local elites to organize epidemic exorcism rites. Magistrates actively participated in the offering rites to local plague gods (*wenshen jiao*) and the accompanying boat exorcism rituals (*wenchuan*; see Katz 1990: 198–99). In 1748, when an epidemic spread through Hunan, Governor-General Xin Zhu ordered local officials to donate medicine and food to victims, but he also ordered that they increase their efforts in appealing to the plague gods (*GZD I*, Xin Zhu memorial, Qianlong 13/10/9 [1748], group 4, doc. 207.9).

In the late nineteenth century, exorcism rituals continued to be a central aspect of epidemic relief. Paul Katz (1991: 16–17) describes how, late in the century, magistrate for Yongjia county (in Zhejiang) presented a memorial to the Emperor of Heaven asking that an epidemic be stopped. Similarly, Wu Dacheng, the Hunan governor in 1893, undertook the following measures after an epidemic struck the county of Anren: "I respectfully composed a written message to the gods, and sent an official forward to each place to sincerely worship the plague gods of each, and to extend respectful prayers to heaven for heavenly protection. After this, the epidemic gradually subsided and the people were greatly consoled" (*GZD II*, Wu Dacheng memorial, Guangxu 19/11/18 [1893], group 359-4-75, box no. 92).

Although local officials tried to prevent epidemic outbreaks through prayer and ritual, in the material realm the state's response was largely crisis-oriented. Official efforts at epidemic prevention were limited to repairing and cleaning up public thoroughfares, getting rid of rubbish, and burning the clothing and personal belongings of victims after an epidemic broke out. Significantly, with the exception of measures implemented in the Imperial Court against smallpox, prior to the twentieth century the Qing government did not attempt to prevent epidemic disease through the use of quarantine or the isolation of victims (Chang 1993; Leung 1987: 142).

The lack of state-imposed quarantine can be accounted for in a number of ways. Angela Leung suggests that Confucian normative values acted against segregating the sick and that the state condemned families who abandoned their relatives during epidemics (Leung 1987: 144). This value was reinforced by the popular belief that the gods would only spare those filial enough to honor their parents. Moreover, she argues, even if the will to impose quarantine had existed, it is doubtful that the imperial Chinese state had the ability to carry out what were fundamentally coercive measures requiring extensive bureaucratic management and policing powers.

While Leung is correct in her assessment that both moral values and practical difficulties inhibited the use of quarantine in China, she deemphasizes another important factor: Chinese medical conceptions about the etiology of infectious disease. Leung argues that neither Chinese nor premodern European medical theory stressed contagion as the primary cause of plague. As the discussion earlier in this chapter has shown, this was certainly true of Chinese medicine. In practical terms, the Chinese seem to have recognized that some diseases were contagious because households posted notices on their gates and placed the dying out on the street. Nonetheless, this was not a part of any classical medical doctrine. Since the concept of direct contagion was not widely accepted among physicians in China, there was little medical rationale for the segregation of patients.

Yet there was more controversy in early modern Europe over the etiology of infectious disease than Leung's analysis implies. Beginning with classical Greek medicine, the Western tradition has always had theorists who believed that diseases such as plague were contagious (Nutton 1983: 1–34). Even during those eras when contagionism was not in the mainstream of medical thought, it influenced public policy (Carmichael 1986: 127–31). In the late medieval period, Italian city-states devised quarantine, *lazaretto* (pest houses), and local health boards to control the spread of plague—measures based on the assumption that plague spread directly from person to person (ibid.: 192–200). By the sixteenth and seventeenth centuries, these measures were widely used in northern Europe as well.

Although official reportage on epidemics is very sparse, the few memorials that do exist show little variation across time or space in the strategies Qing officials used to deal with epidemic disease: for the most part, officials simply distributed medicine to the stricken area. With the exception of smallpox outbreaks that threatened the Court directly, the state did not seek to prevent epidemics by imposing quarantine. This does not mean that the Chinese government was indifferent to the suffering brought on by disease. Local officials responded as best they could, using the strategies of charitable relief, cleanup campaigns, appeals to the plague gods, and participation in community ceremonies and processionals. In short, during the eighteenth and nineteenth centuries, the state had a relatively limited repertoire for dealing with the plague epidemics that were affecting so many communities in southern China.

Conclusion

Concepts of disease are always mediated by language and culture, and every society frames disease in its own way (Rosenberg 1992: xiii–xxvi). The trauma of the fourteenth century Black Death haunted Europeans for centuries, and "plague," the reputed cause of the medieval disaster, came to serve not only as the name of a specific disease but as a generic label for any form of pestilence and as a metaphor for the total disintegration of the individual and society as well (Herzlich and Pierret 1987: 39). Similarly, the Arabic designation for plague, ta'un, had both the generic sense of "an epidemic" and the specific meaning of plague (Dols 1977: 315). In contrast, in China the disease now known to be caused by the *Yersinia pestis* bacteria remained unnamed by a specific term until the late nineteenth century. These different naming strategies highlight how the verbal constructions of "plague" reflect the particular perceptions of a given culture.

Although concepts of disease are socially constructed, many afflictions, including plague, are nonetheless biological events that affect all human bodies in roughly the same way. In the era before antibiotics, plague was a highly fatal disease and few who contracted it survived. Death came quickly, but not before several days of intense suffering. The tender, swollen lymph nodes that marked the onset of the bubonic form were excruciatingly painful; high fevers, delirium, and internal bleeding soon followed. On the fourth or fifth day, the victim went into shock and died. Plague's lethality and its brutal pathogenesis must have made it an extremely frightening and horrific disease in any cultural context.

These stark biological facts about plague pathology meant that individual residents and communities faced common dilemmas during epidemic outbreaks regardless of historical or geographical location. Scholars who have studied past plague epidemics in Europe and the Middle East have been impressed with the similarity of social and intellectual responses across cultures and across time. In what Richard Evans has described as the "common dramaturgy" of epidemics, many people in plague-stricken areas panic and flee (Slack 1992: 3). Carriers of disease are identified and scapegoats found, generally foreigners or members of outcast groups. Believers seek spiritual solace and divine intervention; the sick cast about for miracle cures.

Given that the Chinese faced the same biological event in the eighteenth and nineteenth centuries that people in Europe and the Middle East had earlier, it is not surprising to find that they responded in these ways as well.[38] Lacking any effective practical measure against plague, Christians, Muslims, Buddhists, and Daoists all sought spiritual assistance, and community leaders organized prayers, processionals, and exorcistic rituals designed to lift the scourge. In both Europe and China, plague was seen by many as a sign of divine wrath for lack of human piety or for immoral behavior. In either case, public demonstrations of prayer and repentance were considered proper responses. In Europe, many showed their sincerity through self-flagellation; in China, spirit mediums would injure themselves in part to display the repentance of the community as a whole. In China, as in Europe, one explanation for the appearance of an epidemic was that excessive behaviors (too much food, drink, sexual activity) had displeased the gods (or God). Many people gave up eating meat or abstained from sex as a form of repentance, and private citizens engaged in good works and charitable relief in order to save themselves and their communities.

Through practical experience, people in all three cultural areas knew that plague was linked in some way to the environment and that large numbers of rats always died before the outbreak of human disease. Some unknown force in the atmosphere seemed to be responsible for this phenomenon. European and Islamic medicine located the source of these epizootics and subsequent human epidemics in the malodorous air that arose from decaying matter. The broad outlines of the Warm Factor tradition's etiological theory were quite similar to this miasmatic interpretation, resulting in the use of parallel treatments and preventive measures. Until the eighteenth century, when plague finally disappeared from Europe, a common prophylactic measure was to wear amulets filled with medicaments around the neck or wrist (Baldwin 1993: 227–47). The Chinese also carried satchels filled with herbal remedies that they held under their noses to ward off disease. Both Chinese and Europeans set bonfires during epidemics to clear out poisonous vapors thought to issue from polluted water, rubbish, and the ground. Following an epidemic outbreak, Chinese, like Europeans and Arabs, swept the streets, cleaned around communal wells, and burned the personal effects of plague victims in order to dispel potentially harmful *qi*. Local leaders hastened to bury the dead lest corpses become new sources of putrefaction and disease.

Public health administration was the one area in which Chinese reactions to epidemic disease differed greatly from European reactions. In contrast to Europe, where government-imposed quarantines directly affected people's lives, the imperial Chinese state did not impose forceful public-health measures, partially because it was institutionally unable to do so and partially because Chinese medical theory did not include the idea of direct contagion. This was to change, however, as Western concepts of state medicine began to be accepted and adopted within China. As the next two chapters demonstrate, this shift in state policy was greatly influenced by the international politics of health engendered by the third pandemic of plague.

CHAPTER 5

Civic Activism, Colonial Medicine, and the 1894 Plague in Canton and Hong Kong

PLAGUE ERUPTED in China at a time when the empire was undergoing monumental social and political change. Chinese society was by no means inert before 1800, but in the nineteenth century the pace of change increased as both foreign military pressures and domestic instability intensified. The Opium War of 1839–42 forced China open to Western imperialism and resulted in an unprecedented foreign presence in China's cities. A number of mid-century rebellions, particularly the destructive Taiping Rebellion of the 1850's and 1860's, severely undermined the Qing state's control over elite society. Although local luminaries had long involved themselves in the provision of social welfare, often with the encouragement of state policy, the post-Taiping period saw an increase in, and expansion of, the managerial activity of what Mary Rankin (1986) has termed the "extra-bureaucratic activist elite." In the second half of the nineteenth century, merchants and landed gentry formed new-style philanthropic corporations that not only provided charitable relief to their local communities but also served as the locus for autonomous political power. Rankin shows that this trend began with the *shantang* (benevolent associations) movement in the immediate post-Taiping decades. She argues that these charitable agencies often played a central role in local politics and community affairs that went well beyond their formally defined function of philanthropic activity, and she illustrates how activist elite were involved in public management of all kinds — military, philanthropic, religious, educational, and fiscal (Rankin 1986: 202–47; see also Esherick and Rankin 1990: 334–38).

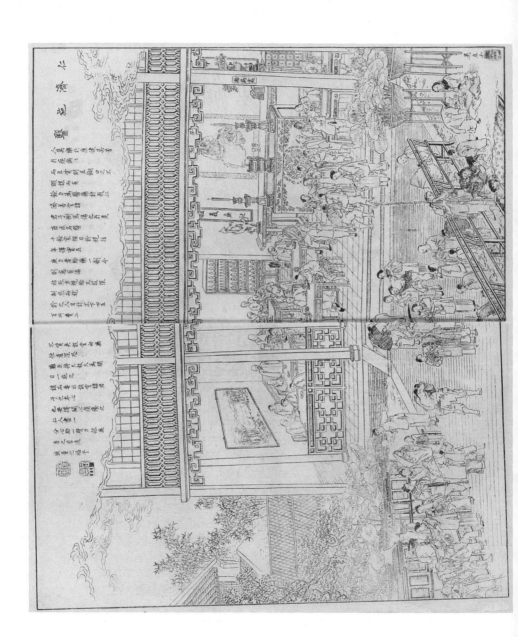

By the time plague appeared in the Pearl River Delta in the 1890's, these transformations were well underway. Hong Kong, ceded to the British by the Treaty of Nanjing in 1842, had been a colony for more than fifty years. Foreigners had taken up residence not only in Canton but in inland areas of Guangdong as well. Elite-initiated *shantang* were flourishing in both Canton and Hong Kong. It was these elite philanthropic associations that directed relief efforts when both cities were struck by plague in 1894. In Canton, Qing officials did not oppose, and may have even supported, such extrabureaucratic initiatives in public health work. In contrast, the British colonial government in Hong Kong sought to curb Chinese elite management of the crisis. The story of how Cantonese *shantang* responded to the 1894 plague underscores the importance of Chinese elite activism in municipal governance at the end of the nineteenth century. The history of plague in Hong Kong during the same year illustrates how this civic response was at odds with the emerging European doctrine of state medicine, as implemented in Britain's Chinese colony.

Civic Activism in Canton:
Shantang Respond to the Plague

The emergence of new types of corporate elite organizations in Guangdong province in the post-Taiping period typifies the late-nineteenth-century civic activism described by Rankin (1986). In Canton, the period between 1870 and 1900 saw the establishment of nine large merchant-directed philanthropic institutions and many smaller ones (*Nanhaixian zhi* 1910, 6: 10b–13a; *Panyuxian xu zhi* 1931, 5: 27–29). The *Aiyu shantang* (called the "Chinese Dispensary" by foreign residents) was the oldest of these halls, having been established in 1871 (*Nanhaixian zhi* 1910, 6: 10b–11a). Its functions were typical of the other benevolent societies in the city and included providing coffins for the poor, distributing free medicine to the sick, and comforting the dying (Figure 11). The charitable halls were financed principally by merchants, and their directorates were made up of merchant-elite (Lum

---

FIG. 11 (*opposite*). "Medical charity of the Renji *shantang*." A nineteenth-century woodcut illustrating the free clinic of the Renji *shantang*. The text notes that because of certain financial difficulties imposed on the *shantang* by this charitable activity, the clinic was open only every other day. From *Dianshizhai huabao* 1983 [1885] 4/*ding*.12: 92. Courtesy of the Library of Congress.

1985: 116–96; Rhoads 1974: 104). It was these recently established corporate charities that coordinated the communal response to plague in Canton.

The 1894 plague epidemic began in Canton as early as February, but there was no public notice of the outbreak until a Chinese-language newspaper mentioned it on March 14 (Sinn 1989: 159).[1] The same article noted that officials had ordered street cleaning (Inspectorate General, *Customs Medical Reports* 1894, no. 48: 20). On April 11, officials again issued a proclamation that the streets be cleaned and that all rubbish be thrown into the river rather than sold (Niles 1894: 116). About twenty coolies were hired to clean up the city. The population was reminded of a regulation that all night soil be taken away before ten o'clock in the morning and that it always be carried in covered buckets.[2] Notices were posted against the slaughter of pigs and against fishing in the river; the authorities also mandated that the clothing of plague victims be burned (*NCH* May 18, 1894: 774). As part of their general efforts to clean up the city during the epidemic, several officials offered rewards for the collection of dead rats (Niles 1894: 116). Coolies then carried these outside the city and buried them.

Medical relief efforts in Canton beyond these officially mandated measures were conducted primarily by *shantang*. A Chinese newspaper article, translated in the *North China Herald* (the original newspaper is not identified) described the activities of a number of these agencies during the 1894 crisis:[3]

Thanks to the charitable institutions of Canton, which came nobly to the fore—such as the *Jêntsi* [*Renji*], *Kuangtsi* [*Guangji*], *Szemiao* [*Simiao*], etc.—nothing was neglected where there was a chance of saving life. One institution, the *Tungshan* [*Tong shantang*] went further; they engaged a good doctor named Chu, who was put in charge of a quantity of medicines and drugs, and sent along the streets of the suburbs, so that those who lived too far away from the city centre, or were unable to go so far, could apply to Chu for advice and medicines they required. The *Jêntsi*, owing to their own restricted quarters in the city, which is full to overflowing with plague patients, got a very large boat as a floating hospital, which is moored at Ngaochow, opposite Honam, or south of the river. Placards also have been posted calling upon skilful physicians to apply to the charity institutions for regular engagements, the idea being to have so strong a force of medical advisers that should any of these also be stricken down, the usual means may not be straitened for want of them. Moreover, such doctors as stayed at home were called upon to give aid, gratis, at their offices, and then apply to the institutions for remuneration if so desired. (*NCH* June 15, 1894: 946)

The *shantang* also served as hospices for the dying and provided burials for the dead. Mary Niles (1894: 119) reported that at the end of the third month of the epidemic, the *Aiyu shantang* had distributed over three hundred free coffins (the usual number per month was twenty or thirty). Nor were these activities limited to Canton. In Beihai, for example, a Chinese hospital, the *Taihe yiju*, was formed in 1890 by Cantonese merchants, and one of its functions was to care for sojourners during the many plague epidemics that occurred in western Guangdong (Wong and Wu 1935: 343).

In addition to these established institutions, the crisis of plague inspired philanthropists to set up special hospices. Tan Congchan, a Shaozhou man, engaged doctors known for their clinical skill, bought medicine and supplies, and opened a medical facility. So many people came to the clinic in the first week that the medicine was rapidly used up. The doctors became so exhausted that they "climbed over the wall and ran away," and Tan Congchan was forced to hire others. In addition to treating plague patients, the emergency clinic bought land to bury plague victims (*Nanhaixian zhi* 1910, 20: 15b–16b). Other generous elite attempted to stem the epidemic by collecting and disposing of rats. A certain Luo Fang, depicted in Figure 12, offered to buy any dead rats brought to him because he believed that the epidemics raging in Guangdong were caused by the foul *qi* of the rotting corpses. The commentary concludes, "In one day he collected more than one thousand rats. There were countless numbers that he could not collect. No wonder the epidemic could not be stopped" (*Dianshizhai huabao* 1983 [1894] 32/*le*.5: 32).

For foreigners living in Canton, the Chinese response to plague was inadequate precisely because it was organized and directed largely by civic leaders rather than officials. Canton's *shantang* had mobilized against the plague, but in the eyes of many Europeans civic activism alone was not sufficient. From the Western perspective, China lacked the kind of efficient governmental involvement deemed essential to effective epidemic prevention and control. John Kerr, the director of the Canton Missionary Hospital, lamented that in "the great city of Canton, . . . there was no Sanitary Board, the government adopted no sanitary or preventive measures, there was no isolation of cases, no removal of filth or rubbish, no water supply, no system of drainage, and . . . Chinese medicine and Chinese superstitions had full and unrestricted sway" (Kerr 1894: 178).[4] In nearby Hong Kong, Chinese reliance on civic leadership during the 1894 plague epidemic conflicted

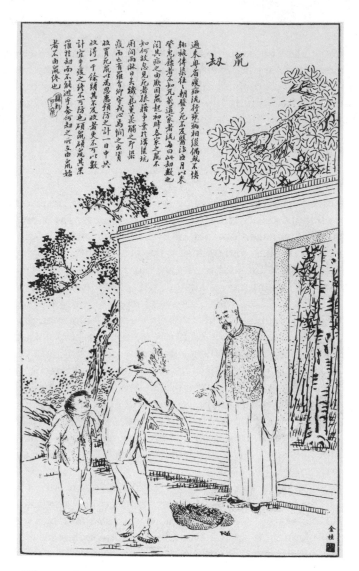

FIG. 12. "The rat disaster." The text of this woodcut refers to the 1894 epidemics in Guangdong and discusses the relationship between the deaths of large numbers of rats and human illness, noting: "In the beginning, the rats of every household died suddenly for no reason at all. Their carcasses were indiscriminately cast into ditches and toilets. After several days' exposure in the rain, the foul *qi* evaporated into the air. Whoever came into contact with this *qi* would immediately contract the disease and die." The text goes on to say that Luo Fang's efforts to stop the epidemic by collecting and disposing of dead animals was futile because "the disaster began with rats but it cannot be ended with them." From *Dianshizhai huabao* 1983 [1894] 32/*le.*5: 31. Courtesy of the Library of Congress.

with late-nineteenth-century Western ideas about the proper role of government in the management of public health concerns.

The Clash Between Civic Activism and State Medicine in Hong Kong

The Donghua Directorate Responds to Plague in Hong Kong

Although Hong Kong was formally governed by the British, informal leadership among the Chinese living in the colony rested with a merchant-elite-managed charitable institution known as the Donghua Hospital (*Tung Wah*). Founded in 1872, the Donghua Hospital resembled most other post-Taiping benevolent halls in both form and function (Sinn 1989: 63–64; Tsai 1993: 70–72).[5] The hospital forwarded the corpses of overseas Chinese to their native villages and helped the sick and destitute return home. It ran free schools and organized societies for the protection of women and children. It provided free medicine and vaccinated children against smallpox. In 1879 alone, the hospital admitted more than 1,000 patients, treated some 82,000 outpatients, provided 221 burials, and helped over 100 poor people return to China (Endacott 1958: 187). It differed from other *shantang*, however, in that it was an inpatient hospital as well as a charitable hall (Sinn 1989: 52).

The functions of the Donghua Hospital and its managers were never limited to medicine or charity alone. As with other elite-managed benevolent organizations in the late-Qing period, the board of directors served as a public decision-making body within the Chinese community. Whereas in Chinese cities the managers of *shantang* often mediated between officialdom and the population, in Hong Kong petitions addressed to British authorities were channeled through the Donghua Directorate. The Hong Kong government often chose to consult with the hospital board on matters that affected the Chinese. The managers of the Donghua Hospital were also in close contact with merchant-elite and officials in Canton.

In 1894 the Donghua Hospital Directorate took charge of plague relief efforts among the Chinese residents of Hong Kong (Sinn 1989: 159–83). The board of directors set up a branch hospital for the treatment of plague victims where only classical Chinese therapies were used. No attempt was made to isolate plague patients from their families. The Directorate also sought to assist the sick and dying in returning to China. In this, its activities extended beyond the colony itself. A branch hospital of the Donghua group was established at Lizhijiao (Lai-chi-kok), just across the border on the Kowloon Peninsula (ibid.: 178). Together with the Canton-based *Aiyu shantang*, the board also established the Lizhijiao Cemetery for plague victims (Tung Wah [Donghua] Group of Hospitals, Editorial Board 1961: 102–3). A Kowloon-based *shantang*, the *Le shantang* (Lok-shin-tong), set up a similar cemetery (Hayes 1977: 170).

As the undisputed leaders of the Chinese community, the directors of the hospital thought it natural that they would direct relief efforts in the Chinese sections of Hong Kong during the 1894 plague outbreak there. This placed them in direct conflict with the British colonial government, which increasingly saw state medicine and the sanitary regulation of the Chinese community as among its basic functions. Unlike their counterparts in Canton, the leaders of Hong Kong's *shantang* faced significant governmental opposition to their plague relief efforts.

State Medicine and Public Health Reform in Colonial Hong Kong

State medicine was a concept that developed gradually in Europe and North America over the course of the nineteenth century. Its central tenets were that the state had primary responsibility for protecting the public's health and that it therefore had the right, even the duty, to impose hygiene and sanitation regulations on private citizens for the public good. Early in the century, Western governments were generally involved in public health matters only when epidemics threatened, and this laissez-faire spirit only gradually gave way to more interventionist policies. But by century's end—spurred by the mid-century sanitationist reform movement and the microbiological revolution of the 1880's and 1890's—European and American governments felt increasingly compelled to monitor and manage sanitation and public health concerns on a more consistent basis.

England was in the forefront of the state medical movement, being the first nation to enact centralized public-health legislation (Brand 1965: 5). Before the Industrial Revolution, government management of public health concerns in Britain, as elsewhere, was sporadic, crisis-oriented, and highly localized. As rapid industrialization and urbanization brought overcrowding and increased disease, British reformers began to lobby for greater governmental attention to public health (Fee and Porter 1992). Particularly in the wake of cholera epidemics in the mid-nineteenth century, radical sanitarians such as Edwin Chadwick called for legislative measures to deal with the problem of ill health in England's cities and towns. Despite the efforts of these early reformers, national government action was not taken until the 1860's and 1870's, when the British state medical and public health movements at last began to gain ground (Brand 1965: 7–21). The first truly effective national Sanitary Act was passed in 1866; successive legislation over the next seven years expanded the jurisdiction of the national government over health matters (Duffy 1993: 202). Passage of a comprehensive health law in 1875 finally established an extensive national public-health system in Britain.

Inspired by the legislation passed in England in the 1870's, sanitarians in Hong Kong urged the colonial authorities there to expand regulation and oversight of public health matters, not only in the European settlement but in the broader Chinese districts as well. Debate had already existed for years over the extent to which the colonial government should impose Western-style public health measures on Chinese residents (Endacott 1958: 183–88, 199–202; Sinn 1989: 160). Since the 1840's the Hong Kong authorities had followed the enclavist impulses that informed British colonial administration in India and elsewhere (Arnold 1993: 96–98), maintaining a policy of nonintervention in health matters that did not affect Europeans (Endacott 1958: 199–202). Public health laws had been passed but were not for the most part acted upon.

Frustrated by government inaction in Hong Kong, sanitarians continued to lobby for public health reform throughout the 1870's. Based on their belief that infectious disease was caused primarily by miasmas arising from unsanitary environments, these reformers were appalled at the smells, the overcrowding, and the "filth" of Chinese dwellings. Successive colonial surgeons urged the Hong Kong government to clean up unsightly and "odorous" neighborhoods. Ammunition for their cause was provided by Osbert Chadwick, Edwin Chadwick's son, who visited Hong Kong in 1882 and produced a report on the sanitation conditions of the colony in which he recommended vigorous and fundamental changes in governmental policy (Sinn 1989: 250).

As a consequence of these mounting pressures for reform, the Hong Kong government established a permanent Sanitary Board in 1883. The Board was given wide powers in theory, including the rights to inspect private residences, disinfect premises deemed unsanitary, and remove contagious persons to isolation hospitals. In practice, however, the Board's powers were blocked over the next decade by opponents who continued to advocate an enclavist approach in matters of public health. Much of the opposition came from landlords, both Chinese and European, who feared that measures designed to reduce overcrowding and clean up their properties would be too costly. There was also genuine sympathy for the hardship such measures would cause the poor, as well as a pragmatic recognition that stringent policies would provoke such opposition among Chinese residents as to make enforcement impossible (Choa 1981: 71–89). Moreover, through the 1880's the colonial government was largely content to leave management of the Chinese sectors of the city in the hands of the elite corporate leadership in Hong Kong—namely, the Donghua Hospital Directorate.

Plague Policies of the Hong Kong Government

The plague epidemic of 1894 offered an opportunity to those who advocated greater public-health monitoring of Chinese neighborhoods.[6] The outbreak seemed to prove the sanitarians correct because the disease tended to appear in conditions of overcrowding and dirt, particularly in the poorer Chinese districts. When Alexandre Yersin and Kitasato Shibasaburo independently isolated the plague bacillus in Hong Kong in 1894, the reformers had what they believed was concrete microscopic evidence of the dangers arising from the habits and living conditions of the Chinese (Hirst 1953: 106–7). As noted in a paper published in the *Journal of the American Medical Association* in 1894, "The malady is undoubtedly a filth disease and is caused by a bacillus. It has been named 'the disease of barbarism,' from the fact that it only occurs among the semi-civilized" (Foster 1894: 7).

Although Yersin and Kitasato identified the plague bacterium in 1894, Western medical theory had not yet determined that bubonic plague is a rat-flea-borne disease. Moreover, because for many years there was no consensus in Western medical circles about how plague is transmitted, physicians and administrators in Hong Kong held conflicting theories about how the bacillus spread. At an 1896 meeting of the British Medical Association of Hong Kong, for example, some participants speculated that the disease was transmitted through the alimentary tract, while others believed that it came from a miasmal vapor ("Infection in Bubonic Plague" 1896: 54). The dominant model in the minds of colonial officials was a blend of contagionist and environmentalist thinking. Many believed that bubonic plague was a directly contagious disease caused by overcrowding and inattention to basic hygiene on the part of Chinese residents. For example, an anonymous article in the *China Medical Missionary Journal* describes a paper that Dr. James Lowson presented at the 1896 British Medical Association meeting in Hong Kong, in which he argued that the plague bacillus "multiplies" in the human body and in the dust found in unclean dwellings, and also noted that infection occurred when one came into contact either with contagious Chinese or with their surroundings (ibid.).

Others believed that the disease was not directly contagious but could be contracted from the personal effects of Chinese residents. W. E. Hunt, the American consul in Hong Kong, articulated the belief that plague was transmitted via the living space of the Chinese:[7]

The disease is still supposed to be non-contagious, and does not take the form of an epidemic to which all nationalities are equally liable, it having proved to be contagious only when one is thrown directly in to contact with the disease and is surrounded with the unspeakable filth in which thousands of the natives have lived in utter indifference to sanitary laws.

The American consul in Canton also pursued this line of thought:[8]

I am persuaded that with the observance of proper precautions, especially in assuring the supply of pure water for cooking and washing, and for flushing drains in times of drouth; there should be no such thing as this "Plague," except where natives in congested localities cause pollution of the air by overcrowding and filth, and violation of sanitary conditions for safety.

Even after 1898, when Paul Simond published his classic paper hypothesizing that the rat flea was the missing link in the chain of plague transmission, many Western authorities initially refused to accept it (Hirst 1953: 152–63). When laboratory studies in Hong Kong failed to demonstrate that rats could be infected by fleas, scientists concluded that "plague infected fleas are of no practical importance in regard to the spread of plague" (ibid.: 159), and authorities thus continued to believe that plague was spread by direct contact either between people or with their household items.

Given that many Western scientists and officials thought that the bubonic form of plague was a contagious "filth" disease, the anti-plague policies of the Hong Kong authorities centered on the apprehension and control of Chinese residents and on the destruction of their homes or personal belongings. After the first reports of plague in Hong Kong, the colonial government quickly took steps to strengthen the Sanitary Board. A permanent committee was set up and bylaws were passed that enlarged its powers considerably. The Sanitary Board

Comparison of Plague-Specific Death Rates and Case-Fatality Rates Between
the Chinese and Non-Chinese Population of Hong Kong, 1894–1907

Year	Chinese plague deaths per 1,000	Non-Chinese plague deaths per 1,000[a]	Chinese case-fatality rate	Non-Chinese case-fatality rate
1894	10.84	3.82	95.88%	68.33%
1895	0.15	0.00	83.72	0.00
1896	4.51	2.63	90.49	65.96
1897	0.08	0.00	90.48	0.00
1898	4.75	3.39	90.51	64.47
1899	5.85	1.35	97.11	67.74
1900	4.10	0.98	—[b]	—[b]
1901	5.73	2.81	93.34	—[b]
1902	1.88	1.04	98.72	76.92
1903	4.02	2.32	93.20	35.54
1904	1.51	0.16	96.65	100.00
1905	0.81	0.16	94.67	75.00
1906	2.69	0.74	94.94	69.57
1907	0.62	0.25	82.48	83.33
Average (1894–1907):	3.40	1.40		
Average (not including 1900–1901):			92.40%	58.91%

SOURCE: Hong Kong Government 1894–1908, *Hong Kong Legislative Council Sessional Papers.*
[a]Non-Chinese population included Europeans, Indians, Japanese, Filipinos, Eurasians, Portuguese, Malays, and West Indians.
[b]Number of cases not reported.

authorized troops stationed in the colony to conduct house-to-house searches and remove all plague victims or corpses. Persons suspected of having plague were taken to a hospital ship, the *Hygeia*; the dead were buried on the outskirts of the city in mass graves. At the height of the epidemic, the central area of Victoria (the Taipingshan district) was cordoned off, streets were walled up, and guards were stationed around the perimeter.

This intensified level of intervention by the colonial government in Hong Kong was precipitated less by any real threat the disease posed to the European community than by fear that the epidemic would spread to the European enclave from Chinese neighborhoods.[9] Although plague killed more than twenty-five hundred people in Hong Kong during 1894, few Europeans became infected, a fact evident from government statistics collected between 1894 and 1907 (Table 20; see also Appendix A). Not only did fewer foreigners contract the disease, they were less likely to die from it than were Chinese residents. Whereas case-fatality rates for Chinese victims in Hong Kong ranged from 82 to 99 percent, those for non-Chinese living in the colony exceeded 80 percent only in 1904 and 1907, when the total number of cases among non-Chinese was below ten. On average, 92 percent of all Chinese who contracted plague died of it, compared to an average of 59 percent of infected non-Chinese over the same period of time.[10]

Because bubonic plague is a rat-flea-borne disease and rats do thrive in unsanitary surroundings, there was a biological foundation for European observations that the epidemic was most virulent in poorer, more densely populated neighborhoods, where solid waste disposal was presumably a problem. Limited information on the social geography of plague outbreaks in Hong Kong between 1894 and 1907 bears out the observation that the poor were indeed the most afflicted. In 1894 the Kennedytown district of Hong Kong was by far the worst affected when plague broke out, with 66 percent of the total reported deaths in the colony (Hong Kong Government, *Blue Book Reports on Bubonic Plague* 1895: 158–59, 390–91). Ten percent of the total recorded deaths occurred in Taipingshan, and 9 percent in Xiyingpang (Saiyingpun; ibid.). Over the fourteen-year period between 1894 and 1907, 20 percent of all reported plague deaths occurred in Kennedytown (Table 21). These districts were the most densely populated areas of Victoria and were those where poor migrant laborers tended to live (Leeming 1977: 58–60).

Although European fears of the Chinese underclass and their "lack of hygiene" had some basis in fact, the point here is that public policy was driven less by a clear sense of plague etiology than by incomplete knowledge combined with preconceived notions about Chinese habits. Colonial authorities assumed that plague was a contagious "filth" disease, and they therefore expected it to appear in the bodies and houses of the poor. It followed that the proper course of action was to undertake a sanitizing campaign in these poor districts, to detain victims, and to maintain the strict segregation between "natives" and Europeans. While efforts to clean up the houses and clothing of Chinese residents may have destroyed some rats and fleas, it was not yet known that eradication campaigns had to target these vectors directly in order to be truly effective. As a consequence, there was no demonstrable lessening of the epidemic in the colony even after anti-plague policies were put into effect.

TABLE 21

Distribution of Plague in Districts of Hong Kong and Kowloon, 1894–1907

District	No. of plague deaths in each district	Percentage of total plague deaths in each district
City of Victoria		
Sokonpo	369	2.95
Bowrington	918	7.34
Wanchai	156	1.25
Hawan	736	5.89
Sheungwan	683	5.46
Chungwan	540	4.32
Taipingshan	729	5.83
Xiyingpang	769	6.15
Shektongtsui	1,314	10.51
Kennedytown	2,520	20.15
Victoria Peak	22	0.18
Unknown	158	1.26
Subtotal	9,672	77.34
Victoria harbor	614	4.91
Kowloon		
Land	1,492	11.93
Boat	234	1.87
Shaukiwan		
Land	134	1.07
Boat	12	0.15
Aberdeen		
Land	43	0.34
Boat	3	0.02
Stanley		
Land	6	0.05
Boat	0	
Foreign community	296	2.37
TOTAL	12,506	100.00

SOURCE: Hong Kong Government 1894–1908, *Hong Kong Legislative Council Sessional Papers.*

Chinese Resistance to Plague Policies in Hong Kong

The Donghua Hospital Directorate organized opposition to British antiplague measures, particularly the government's mandatory house-to-house inspection campaign, its policy of forced hospitalization, and its efforts to prevent plague patients from leaving the colony. On May 20, 1894, Liu Weichuan (Lau Wai Chuen), a prominent member of the Directorate, chaired a large meeting at the hospital attended by seventy members of leading firms, about four hundred other people, the superintendent of police, and the colonial surgeon at Donghua Hospital (Sinn 1989: 167). The main item on the agenda was the Hong

Kong government's refusal to allow plague victims to leave the colony. Liu Weichuan suggested that the leading Hong Kong firms petition the governor to rescind the strict quarantine on emigration, and this was agreed upon unanimously (ibid.: 166).

With the population nearing a boiling point, the Hong Kong government backed off from some of the harsher requirements it had proposed. The government agreed not to force patients onto the hospital ship. Instead, they were taken to the "Glass Works" factory at Kennedytown, where a Chinese-style hospital had been set up under Donghua supervision. But these concessions were not sufficient to stem the exodus: an estimated eighty thousand people left Hong Kong during the epidemic (Hong Kong Government, *Blue Book Reports on Bubonic Plague* 1894: 286). Those who remained attempted to hide their sick friends and relatives from the Sanitary Board inspectors (ibid.: 165).

In Canton, anger at the intrusive measures in effect in Hong Kong took the form of placard campaigns against the Hong Kong government.[11] Beginning in late May, some posters warned people not to return to Hong Kong; others reported highly exaggerated rumors about the plague control measures being used in the colony; and still others urged a general uprising against all foreigners living in the Canton area, and against the Chinese government for allowing the Hong Kong government to carry out the plague control measures in the first place. The placards stated that foreigners were dispensing poison in the form of amulets and that foreign missionaries and their assistants were distributing these scent-bags around the city; they also called upon the populace to exterminate all foreigners.

Local English newspapers implied that the Donghua Directorate was behind the placards, an accusation believed by, and enraging to, Hong Kong Governor William Robinson (governed 1891–98). Robinson telegraphed Byron Brenan, the British consul in Canton, insisting that he apply pressure on Li Hanzhang, the governor-general of Guangdong and Guangxi. Following meetings with Brenan, Li Hanzhang issued a proclamation describing conditions in Hong Kong and stating that all patients on the *Hygeia* had either been moved to Donghua Hospital or given passage back to China (Sinn 1989: 172). These statements were actually not true, but they mirrored demands that the Donghua group had been making to the British governor. In fact, Li Hanzhang was "simply transmitting the message of the Hospital Committee which, in desperation, had appealed to the Canton authorities for help" (ibid.: 173). Li Hanzhang offered to send ships to Hong Kong to pick up plague patients and bring them back to Canton. Robinson finally agreed to let plague patients leave the colony on June 9, after he was petitioned by the compradors of several large firms (ibid.: 174–75). The promised boats, apparently chartered by Donghua Hospital, arrived the next day. Ironically, Robinson gave in on the one policy—enforcement of a strict *cordon sanitaire*—that might have prevented the spread of plague to other communities.

Nor did Robinson's concession ameliorate antiforeign sentiment in Canton. When new sanitation measures were introduced in Hong Kong, including a provision that allowed the colonial government to turn people out of their houses and destroy the Taipingshan district, placards again appeared in Canton threatening to burn down the foreign concessions if the neighborhood was razed as planned. Despite these protests, the colonial authorities carried out the proposed cleanup campaign. Some three hundred fifty houses were torn down, and about seven thousand Chinese displaced from their homes. Many more had to stay in temporary shelters for nine days while a process of disinfection was carried out.[12]

On June 11, two American missionary women who were attempting to treat plague victims were attacked by a mob in Canton.[13] After the consuls of Britain, the United States, France, and Germany all protested to Li Hanzhang, he ordered military officers to tear down all posters and arrest any troublemakers. He also asked the foreign consuls to instruct missionaries not to provoke assaults by providing medical aid in Chinese neighborhoods. When Li Hanzhang then wrote to the Zongli Yamen in Beijing, blaming the Hong Kong government for the disturbances, tensions between the British and Chinese over the antiplague measures in Hong Kong threatened to become an international incident (Sinn 1989: 176).

Curtailment of the Donghua Directorate

The 1894 plague in Hong Kong brought into conflict two systems of medical thought, neither of which was particularly effective against bubonic plague. This lack of efficacy created fertile soil for mutual recriminations between advocates of each system, since each could point to the demonstrated failures of the other. Not surprisingly, this pattern of mutual accusation played into deeply held stereotypes of each community. Europeans vilified the Chinese for filth, overcrowding, and unsanitary conditions, while the Chinese viewed Europeans,

and particularly the Hong Kong authorities, as inhumane and fundamentally hostile to Chinese values.

The gulf between European advocacy of state medicine and the atti-
tude of many Chinese is apparent in an editorial that appeared in a
Cantonese newspaper:

As for Hongkong, the plague there is being dealt with solely by the foreign
officials. A friend who arrived at Canton from that island yesterday, spoke of
the enormous number of fatalities there, and the foreign methods of dealing
with the plague, which appear to us ridiculous enough. He said that when a
person is stricken with the plague at Hongkong the foreign officials take them
to the floating hospital moored in the mid-stream. First they make the patient
swallow 12 oz. of brandy, mixed with some kind of liquid medicine. Then they
put six pounds of ice on top of the patient's head, while the chest, hands and
feet are also loaded with a pound of ice each. In this manner not one person
out of ten manages to leave that floating hospital alive. Searchers are also sent
during the day time into the various dwelling-houses and if they happen to
see some one in a recumbent position or taking a nap, down he is pounced
upon as having been plague-stricken, and the unlucky person is forcibly taken
to the floating hospital where with the remedies above mentioned his life is
soon taken away. In this way numberless persons have met an undeserved
fate. (translated in *NCH* June 15, 1894: 946)

Such fears of foreign hospitals were not merely hyperbolic: there was
a 90 percent case-fatality rate in these clinics.[14] Many European physicians readily admitted that there was little they could do to treat
plague other than incise the buboes, ply the patient with alcoholic
"stimulants" (usually brandy or champagne), reduce the fever with ice
compresses, and administer carbolic acid to try to drive out the "blood
poison" (Inspectorate General, *Customs Medical Reports* 1894, No. 48:
51–52, 72). In sum, turn-of-the-century Western plague remedies were
no more efficacious than were classical Chinese therapies.

Despite the dismal record of Western doctors in treating the disease,
many foreigners living in Hong Kong believed that Chinese resistance
to Western medicine was inspired by xenophobic superstition. Moreover, they blamed the Donghua Hospital Directorate for stirring up
popular resistance to plague control measures. As one editorial writer
in the *North China Herald* put it:

Many of the leading Chinese in Hongkong . . . have an idea that the city of
Victoria is almost a Chinese city. . . . These men do their best to stop any regulations being put into force which are repugnant to Chinese ideas, and they
can immediately get up a strike or riot among the lower classes of their fellow
countrymen if the Government does not listen to them. (*NCH* June 1, 1894: 838)

Critics demanded that Donghua Hospital be closed, citing the high case-fatality rates of its plague patients. The governor was also harshly criticized for giving in to the Donghua Directorate's request that plague victims be allowed to leave the colony.

In 1896 a commission was set up to inquire into the work of Donghua Hospital. In its report the commission recommended that the hospital be allowed to remain open but that it be supervised by a Chinese doctor trained in Western medicine, that patients be allowed to choose between Chinese and Western medical treatment, and that it be subject to supervision by the government's medical officer. The rationale for restricting the hospital's activities rested partially on Western disapproval of customary Chinese modes of medical treatment. More fundamentally, the civic activism of the Donghua Hospital Directorate was at odds with the emerging system of state medicine, which held that the government should regulate public health matters.

The Donghua Hospital Directorate attempted to retain some degree of autonomy in subsequent years, and it continued to mediate between the government and Chinese residents during outbreaks of plague. In 1901, for example, in a letter to the Hong Kong registrar-general, it conveyed the complaints of Chinese residents that antiplague disinfection efforts damaged their household goods and clothing. The Donghua group proposed that its directors supervise the sterilization process to ensure that it was done carefully (Sinn 1984: 217). But the hospital's activities had come under close governmental scrutiny and its power, even in medical matters, was vastly curtailed. When, in 1901, the Canton *Aiyu shantang* asked the Directorate for help in getting the British government to remove restrictions on the movement of plague victims, the Directorate replied that it had no influence over the Colonial Office. It suggested instead that the *Aiyu shantang* rally all the charitable institutions in Canton to petition the governor of Guangdong to ask the British consul in Canton to forward such a request to the Colonial Office (ibid.).

Conclusion

In the decades before 1894, foreign advocates of state medicine and public health reform had been waging a campaign to convince the Hong Kong authorities to actively regulate sanitation among Chinese living in the colony. Full implementation of intrusive Western-style public health measures had been blocked both by Chinese community leaders and by Hong Kong government officials who recognized the opposition such measures would generate among the Chinese population. When the plague epidemics seemed to prove the advocates of sanitation reform correct, the government hastily enacted strict epidemic-control measures, including police inspections, isolation wards, and public health blockades. This was a forceful introduction of colonial state medicine into China, and it met with both popular and elite resistance.

Despite European suspicions to the contrary, conflict between the Hong Kong government and the Chinese community over the plague measures was not simply symptomatic of lingering Chinese superstition and resistance to biomedicine. When Western medicine had shown itself to be efficacious, as in the treatment of eye diseases and in Jennerian smallpox vaccinations, many Chinese were extremely responsive (Wong and Wu 1935: 139). As discussed in Chapter 4, Chinese officials were quite eager to buy foreign drugs, such as *awei*, when it appeared that they worked. In the case of plague, Western treatments in the 1890's were simply not very effective. Chinese residents were reacting not only against medical treatment they regarded as absurd, but against highly intrusive state policies, particularly the mandatory house-to-house inspections, the forced hospitalization methods, and the destruction of houses. In this, Chinese resistance to colonial medical policies was little different from that of other colonized peoples, or indeed, of Europeans who rioted when their own governments imposed mandatory quarantines during epidemics.[15]

Somewhat ironically, the state medical movement in Britain had begun with civic activism. The sanitarian and public health movements had been initiated largely by social reformers and activist physicians in the early and mid-nineteenth century. The central state became actively involved in the management of public health only in the 1860's and 1870's. By the 1890's, many Europeans living in Hong Kong and Canton viewed state medicine as an essential marker of modernity. Continued Chinese reliance on civic leadership during the 1894 plague epidemics in Canton and Hong Kong clashed with these new Western ideas about the proper role of government in the management of public health. Yet within twenty years, Western-style public health management and state medicine were being promoted by Qing officials themselves.

CHAPTER 6

Plague and the Origins of Chinese State Medicine in the New Policies Reform Era, 1901-1911

CHINA'S LOSS to Japan in the war of 1894–95 heightened Chinese anxiety over the Qing dynasty's ability to withstand foreign aggression. Outraged by the disastrous terms of the Treaty of Shimonoseki, scholars led by Kang Youwei called for a new, comprehensive program of governmental reform. The Guangxu emperor's efforts to implement such policies in 1898 were quashed by the Empress Dowager Cixi and Qing conservatives. Cixi authorized reforms only after the Boxer Rebellion failed in 1900. By that time many officials in the Qing Court were convinced that China needed to follow the institutional lead of powerful nation-states such as Germany and Japan if the territorial integrity of the Chinese empire was to be maintained. In a sweeping body of initiatives known as the New Policy (*xinzheng*) Reforms, the Qing state abolished the imperial examination system, established new military and police organizations, streamlined the central bureaucracy, and began to rationalize systems of taxation (Ichiko 1980: 375–415; Wright 1968: 24–63). Toward the end of the decade, the central government moved toward constitutionalism, drafting a plan to adopt a national constitution and establish a system of local self-government. In the end, the New Policy Reforms served to undermine both the Qing dynasty and the imperial system itself. Both were swept away when the Republican Revolution broke out in 1911.

As in other policy realms, the issue of sovereignty was a powerful impetus for change in the public health sphere. In the eyes of many Qing officials, ongoing foreign initiatives in public health, particularly the imposition of ship quarantine in China's treaty ports, were affronts to China's national dignity. At the same time, many Chinese intellectuals began to voice the view that state medicine (*guojia yixue*) was essential for national strength and the survival of the Chinese race (Crozier 1968: 59; Dikötter 1992: 111). Immediately after the Sino-Japanese War, Kang Youwei stressed the necessity of state medicine and public health institutions for the continued vitality of the Chinese people in his 1895 "Ten Thousand Word Memorial" (Crozier 1968: 59–60). Throughout the New Policies reform period, editorials appeared in reform-oriented journals urging the government to establish state medicine, Western-style public health reforms, and antiepidemic measures in order to build the nation (*Dongfang zazhi* Sept. 1904, 1.7: 73–76; Apr. 1905, 2.4: 7–10; and June 1905, 2.6: 107–14).

Following the Boxer Rebellion, Qing officials such as Yuan Shikai began to establish Western-style public health institutions as part of the New Policies reform program. Specifically, Qing reformers borrowed the German and Japanese idea that public health and disease-prevention efforts should be directed by the police. From about 1902 on, new-style police departments in some Chinese cities began to use Western-style disease control techniques such as quarantine and isolation hospitals for the treatment of infectious disease. Gradually, a police-directed model of public health emerged in China, shaped by a statist orientation that was international in scope.

One of the first municipalities to establish police-directed public health institutions was the city of Shenyang (Mukden) in southern Manchuria. These institutional arrangements were severely tested when a virulent epidemic of pneumonic plague spread throughout the northeast in the winter of 1910–11. Although a lack of personnel meant that the goal of total state control went largely unrealized, the Shenyang police actively managed many antiepidemic measures during the crisis. These fledgling public-health reforms were cut short by the lack of centralized state control that followed the 1911 Republican Revolution. The early involvement of the police in these activities nonetheless laid a basis for the development of state medical institutions later in the century.

Plague, Ship Quarantine, and the Issue of Sovereignty

The immediate stimulus for late-Qing reforms in the public health arena was the perceived threat to Chinese sovereignty posed by foreign initiatives in ship quarantine. Foreigners working in the Chinese Imperial Customs Service had first imposed quarantine in Shanghai and Xiamen (Amoy) in 1873, after cholera outbreaks were reported in India and Southeast Asia (Wu 1959: 403–5; Yang Shangchi 1990: 25). Similar regulations went into effect in Shantou (Swatow) in 1883 and in Ningbo (Ningpo) in 1884 (Yang Shangchi 1990: 25). When plague erupted in Canton and Hong Kong in 1894, customs superintendents in Shanghai, Shantou, Xiamen, and Ningbo declared all ships entering their harbors subject to quarantine.[1] These measures were employed thereafter whenever plague was determined to be present in a port (Wong and Wu 1935: 360–61; Yang Shangchi 1990: 25). In 1899 the foreign-run Municipal Council of Shanghai further authorized the establishment of a permanent plague quarantine station on Chongbaosha Island near Wusong (Inspectorate General, *Decennial Reports 1892–1901*, 1: 500–501).[2] Similar stations were established that year in the northern ports of Yingkou (Newchwang) and Tianjin (Tientsin), and in the port of Fuzhou (ibid., 1: 37; 2: 579).[3] The quarantine stations inspected passengers and detained them if they were thought to be suffering from plague or other infectious diseases.

Chinese objections to these foreign initiatives were raised on a number of grounds, including the inconvenience such measures posed for travelers, the expense involved, and quarantine's adverse effects on trade. In 1901 Xu Yingkui, the governor-general of Fujian and Zhejiang, requested that the Fuzhou quarantine station be abolished because it was of limited utility and too expensive to maintain.[4] Li Xingrui, who was briefly the governor-general of Jiangxi and Jiangsu in 1904, complained that the quarantine station at Chongbaosha "agitated" merchants and gentry traveling from southern ports and was "an insult to those who travel from afar" (*Dongfang zazhi* Dec. 1904, 1.10: 129–30). After the Chongbaosha station was established near Shanghai, an unnamed official memorialized the Grand Council asking that it be closed because the foreign methods used there were "unusually cruel and sadistic to the point that many people have died."[5]

For persons unaccustomed to Western medical techniques, the procedures followed in the quarantine stations must have been traumatic. To depart from any port under a declared quarantine, Chinese passengers were subjected to bodily inspection and a thorough process of disinfection. After a state-of-the-art disinfecting plant was established in Xiamen in 1901, Carl Johnson, the consular surgeon and acting port health officer, proudly described the procedures followed:[6]

Our disinfecting chamber is twenty feet long, ten feet wide, and eight feet high, making its capacity 1600 cubic feet. It is lined with Portland cement throughout, including the ceiling and the floor. . . . The passengers come early on the morning of the day of sailing, leave their clothing in the undressing room, each is furnished with a suit of clothing belonging to the plant and goes away for a few hours. The clothing they have left is hung in the chamber and exposed to the [formol] gas for six hours. When the six hours have nearly expired the passengers again go to the "Undressing rooms," leave the clothing belonging to us and enter the bath room naked. After bathing, they pass through the "Dressing room" where they receive their own clothing. I shall inspect them when leaving their body clothing in the morning, again after the bath, before they have dressed, and a third time on board to prevent substitution.

Li Xingrui expressed frustration with such inspections, lamenting that:

In the past we made mistakes [allowing quarantine stations to be set up] and now with these petty and aggravating regulations, we must submit to foreign doctors. This festering problem has gotten worse. We must find a way out of this situation. (*Dongfang zazhi*, Dec. 1904, 1.10: 129–30)

As suggested by Li Xingrui's complaint, the overriding objection to the quarantine stations was that they represented yet another example of foreign encroachment on China's sovereignty. Behind official complaints about the bodily inspections endured by Chinese passengers were deep concerns, both figurative and real, about the foreign intrusions such examinations represented.

Yuan Shikai and Police-Directed Public Health

While Qing conservatives sought to eradicate Western public-health institutions in China, some officials, most prominently Yuan Shikai, became convinced that foreign interference in such matters would cease only when China had its own effective system of quarantine. Yuan Shikai began to champion Western-style public health after the Boxer debacle of 1900. Indeed, the first Chinese-run public health service was the Beiyang Sanitary Service that Yuan Shikai set up in Tianjin in 1902 (Inspectorate General, *Decennial Reports* 1892–1901, 2: 581). One of the Sanitary Service's primary functions was to inspect ships and trains for plague-infected passengers and cargo (*Dongfang zazhi* June 1904, 1.4: 44–46).

Yuan Shikai's stated rationale for using Western-style plague control measures had more to do with international politics than it did with concerns over sanitation. Yuan Shikai feared that, left unchecked, the spread of plague would demonstrate that China was incapable of effectively administering its own territory, thus providing an excuse for further foreign intervention. In 1903, when plague reached the northern port of Yingkou, the French and German consuls informed him that they intended to send their own soldiers and doctors to the port to enforce quarantine. Yuan Shikai countered by adding more constables to the sanitary department and by setting up additional isolation and quarantine stations along the coast and along the railroad. After taking this action, he wrote in a memorial, "the armies and consular officials of each country all understood that the Chinese are not negligent in the matter of controlling epidemics but rather exert extra effort. They are completely without excuses [to intervene]" (Yuan Shikai 1971, 6: 1673–75).

The Beiyang Sanitary Service was explicitly modeled on the German and Japanese systems of public health, which were hierarchically organized and bureaucratically managed by the police. German political theorists had first developed the concept of "medical police" in the eighteenth century, when the mercantilist goals of Prussian monarchs had led to a renewed interest in the health and welfare of "the people" (Rosen 1974: 120–58). First conceived of as encompassing all aspects of public health administration, by the mid-nineteenth century "medical police" referred specifically to state agencies that would regulate and administer disease control activities, organize and supervise state medical personnel, and oversee sanitation (ibid.: 143). In practical terms, these responsibilities devolved to the municipal police.

The modernizing regime of Meiji Japan appropriated these German concepts of state medicine and medical policing (Johnston 1987: 234–52). When the Meiji police system was organized in 1874, the police were placed in charge of supervising sanitation and public health affairs. In December 1879 the central government ordered all prefectural governments to form sanitary departments, and in 1886 the Home Ministry put county police forces in charge of enforcing most health and hygiene regulations on a local level.

Just as Qing reformers borrowed other aspects of modern policing from the Germans and the Japanese, they also assumed that public health concerns would be directed by the police.[7] Tianjin's new-style police force directed the Beiyang Sanitary Service, and this arrangement served as a model for regional efforts elsewhere. When activist officials such as Cen Chunxuan and Zhao Erxun established new-style police forces in Sichuan, Guangdong, and Fengtian (Liaoning), they viewed sanitation and disease control as important police functions. The central Guangdong police bureau, for example, was opened in December 1902, and a sanitary board composed of five police officials was established the following March (Wang Jiajian 1984: 71). The new-style police department of Chengdu (established in 1902–3) also sought to regulate sanitary and medical matters, particularly after Zhou Shanpei was appointed in 1906 to the post of bureau director (Stapleton 1993: 198–237).

From 1906 on, the central Qing government attempted to standardize and centralize these provincial-level public health efforts. A central Sanitary Department (*Weisheng si*) had been established in 1905 under the auspices of the new Ministry of Police (later the Ministry of the Interior; see Brunnert and Hagelstrom 1912: no. 346, p. 118). The department was theoretically responsible for overseeing all matters related to national public health, including ship quarantine and epidemic prevention and control, but during the years the Ministry of Police existed, it was largely preoccupied with establishing a modern police force in Beijing.[8] In 1908 the Ministry of the Interior put forward a proposal to establish police-directed sanitary departments in all provincial and local jurisdictions. Under the plan every province was to have a police superintendent (*Jingwu gongsuo*, or Police Daotai) in charge of police work, including sanitation and public health. The Police Daotai system was only gradually established between 1908 and 1911, and it is not clear how many provinces had new-style sanitary departments by 1911.[9] Nonetheless, the goal of establishing an empirewide system of police-directed public health agencies suggests a growing commitment within the Qing bureaucracy to the basic principles of state medicine: that the state had a responsibility to protect the public's health, using whatever means were necessary.

New-Style Police and Plague Control Work, 1910–11

The depth of this commitment to state management of public health matters was demonstrated during the winter of 1910–11, when a virulent epidemic of pneumonic plague spread throughout Manchuria (Nathan 1967; Wu 1926; Wu 1936). This was the first time Chinese police carried out Western-style epidemic control measures such as quarantine and the detention of plague patients, and thus represents an important milestone in the development of China's twentieth-century state medical system.[10]

Epidemiologically, the Manchurian plague epidemic was unrelated to the bubonic plague epidemics of southern China. The origins of the Manchurian plague lay not in Yunnan but in areas of Mongolia and Siberia where the Siberian marmot or tarbagan (*Marmota sibirica*) sustains a natural plague reservoir. Between 1907 and 1910, the value of marmot skins increased threefold because international furriers learned that marmot fur makes excellent imitation sable (Wu 1936: 31). By 1910, long-standing Qing bans on migration to Manchuria were no longer in effect and thousands of Chinese trappers moved into the area, hoping to make their fortunes by selling marmot skins on the world fur market. Unlike Mongol trappers, who avoided sick animals, the new arrivals trapped any animal they could find. Living together in crowded railway hostels, often with the pelts stacked close by, these neophytes unwittingly placed themselves at great risk.

On October 13, 1910, a migrant trapper in Manzhouli developed pneumonic plague. Unlike the bubonic form, which relies on rodent and flea vectors for its transmission to humans, the pneumonic form can be passed directly from one person to another by coughing or sneezing. The disease spread rapidly through the packed hostels and quickly killed some six hundred men. Panicked trappers fled southward, carrying the disease along the new Manchurian railway system to Harbin on October 27, Changchun on December 31, and Shenyang on January 2, 1911.

By the time this deadly form of plague appeared in Shenyang, medical police work was already well underway. The Fengtian (now Liaoning) Provincial Police force was one of the earliest new-style police forces in China, and it attempted to manage public health matters almost from its founding (Wang Jiajian 1984: 92; Yu Yongmin 1989: 193–99). Established in 1902, the force was reinvigorated in 1905 by the Qing reformer Zhao Erxun, who increased the number of officers substantially, raised their salaries, established a police academy, and appointed a police commissioner (Wang Jiajian 1984: 92). He also stressed the public health functions of the police, setting up a Sanitary Division (*Weisheng ke*) to oversee epidemic prevention and control, street cleaning, inspection of food, beverages, and pharmaceuticals, and the supervision of hospitals (*Fengtian tongzhi* 1982 [1934], 144: 3285). These functions were to be carried out not only in the provincial capital but also by the sanitary divisions of local police departments.[11]

Further reforms in police sanitation work were undertaken by Xu Shichang and Xiliang during their respective terms as governor-

general of the Three Eastern Provinces.[12] In 1909 the Fengtian Provincial Police department established two sanitary brigades, each composed of 209 officers and menial laborers (*Fengtian tongzhi* 1982 [1934],
144: 3285–86). The duties of the brigades included draining gutters,
cleaning up public toilets, and managing public wells. In the realm
of preventive medicine and public health, brigade members were to
provide smallpox vaccinations, inspect food and drug products, keep
records on the notifiable diseases in a given locality, conduct health inspections of shops and restaurants, provide medicine to the poor, and
examine corpses for the cause of death. The police role during epidemics was also made clear: they were to inspect the sick and detain
those deemed to be dangerous carriers of disease. By 1911, when the
pneumonic plague epidemic struck Fengtian, there were 218 police
departments in the province, each with a sanitary division. These departments had 687 branch offices and some 19,197 police constables,
all of whom were to include disease control and prevention in their
general duties (Wang Jiajian 1984: 94).[13]

Government officials in Shenyang, forewarned by the extensive
outbreaks of plague in northern Manchuria, established a Plague Prevention Bureau (*Fangyi zongju*) in late December, even before plague
reached the city (Zhang Yuanqi 1911; International Plague Conference
1912: 249–53). The heads of the Commission of the Interior (*Minzheng
si*) and the Commission of Foreign Affairs (*Jiaoshe si*) were the primary coordinators of these efforts.[14] They were joined by the chief of
police, the Police Daotai of Fengtian, the head of the Fengtian Government Hospital, and a Scottish missionary doctor. These six men drew
up plans for plague prevention and control in Shenyang and its en-
virons (Christie 1914: 236). Their planning was given more urgency
after the first plague case was found near the Shenyang train station
on January 2, 1911 (International Plague Conference 1912: 249). Three
days later the first cases of plague were found within the city walls
(*Shengjing shibao* Jan. 8, 1911: 2).

The Plague Prevention Bureau had a police-directed plague control
plan worked out by January 10, when the new regulations and procedures were published in local newspapers (*Shengjing shibao* Jan. 10,
1911: 5). The city was to be divided into seven police districts, each
with its own plague prevention office.[15] Twelve police officers were assigned to each district office, accompanied by two medical doctors and
coolies who served as sanitation attendants, stretcher bearers, ambu-
lance men, carters, and gravediggers. The police were to cordon off

and guard their respective districts, thereby controlling traffic between different parts of the city. Rickshaws, tramways, and carts were to be inspected and disinfected (International Plague Conference 1912: 251); they were then to be given flags to carry to allow them to move from one district to another (ibid.: 461; see also *Shengjing shibao* Mar. 15, 1911: 5). A police guard was to be placed at each of the eight city gates, and the roads outside the city were to be patrolled to prevent people from fleeing the cordoned areas on foot (International Plague Conference 1912: 460). Residents were to wear colored armbands identifying the district they lived in and were to move from one district to another only with a special permit from the police authorities.

The Fengtian Provincial Police drew up specific regulations to be followed by Shenyang police officers (i.e., provincial police working in Shenyang) during their inspections.[16] Inspectors were to wear a band of white cloth on their sleeves, bearing the characters *sou yi* (investigating the epidemic). They were to visit their assigned posts daily, although the hours of inspection were limited to 9 to 11 A.M. and 1 P.M. to midnight. All deaths, cases of plague, and suspected cases were to be reported immediately. They were also to inspect and report on the sanitation conditions of houses visited:[17]

If any house is found dirty, the occupants are to be instructed to clean their premises immediately. If any part of a dwelling is found to be too damp, and the constable considers it to be the cause of offensive odours, the occupants are to be ordered to purchase disinfectants, such as lime, bichloride, or carbolic fluid. . . . When an unsanitary dwelling is found, the police are to notify the chief of the sanitary department who will at once send a constable to order the place cleaned.

Occupants of a house in which someone had died of plague had to display a sign on the door saying so. The chief of police of the nearest police station was to bury the corpse "a safe distance from the city walls, residences, and public thoroughfares."[18] The police were also to prevent anyone from visiting premises where such a death had occurred.

These plague prevention and control measures were announced on January 12, 1911, and the Shenyang police were immediately mobilized to carry out house-to-house visitations. The police also set up six quarantine and isolation stations for people suspected of having plague and for those with whom they had been in contact (*Shengjing shibao* Jan. 29, 1911: 5). Police prohibitions were issued against large gatherings of any kind: theater performances and periodic markets were closed down, as were brothels, barbershops, bathhouses, and second-hand clothing shops (ibid. Jan. 10, 1911: 5; see also Feb. 26, 1911: 5). The chief of police established a citywide curfew, and no one was allowed to venture out at night (to prevent the transport of corpses or the sick under cover of darkness). Lunar New Year's visits were prohibited, and festivals and processionals were not allowed (Christie 1914: 251). The authorities also offered rewards for "turning in" plague patients (*Shengjing shibao* Jan. 10, 1911: 5).

From the observations of Dr. Dugald Christie, the Scottish mission-ary doctor serving on the Plague Prevention Bureau, it is apparent that the Shenyang police did attend to these duties. He noted that, every morning, the sanitary police,

in clean white overalls and masks, started on their rounds, each party to an appointed district. Inns, lodging houses, and tea-houses were visited daily, as well as any locality where plague cases had occurred, other districts every sec-ond day. If a policeman found what seemed to be a suspicious case, he called in the chief of his party. If it was doubtful, a note of it was taken and another call paid some hours later. If it was clearly plague, bearers were summoned and the patient taken straight to the hospital. The district police-station was notified, the inmates of the house conveyed to the nearest isolation station, the bedding of the sick person and other articles burned, and the house disin-fected and put under guard. (Christie 1914: 249)

In the isolation stations, the patients were medically inspected and their temperature and pulse taken daily, "so as to discover fresh cases and secure their early isolation" (International Plague Conference 1912: 462).

Transients and the poor were singled out for special attention by the police. Early in the epidemic, it was clear that a disproportion-ate number of cases occurred among sojourning trappers and migrant laborers:[19]

For certain classes of the community, such as beggars and waifs, and for immi-grants, *segregation stations* were instituted. For this purpose empty warehouses, railway cars, or rapidly erected wooden barracks were employed, mostly in the form of large wards. The cases of plague were largely restricted to the coolie class and the lowest orders. (International Plague Conference 1912: 462)

Common prostitutes were also inspected regularly (*Shengjing shibao* Mar. 7, 1911: 5).

Despite the provincial authorities' voiced commitment to using the police to manage the antiepidemic measures, the Plague Prevention Bureau lacked adequate financing and personnel to carry out all its goals effectively. The plan called for trained medical inspectors to take charge of each of the seven police districts. But there were simply not enough doctors available for the task, and medical students, some in their first years of medical school, were substituted (NCH Feb. 10, 1911: 293). Finding men to serve as assistants to the doctors was even more difficult: many of those hired soon died of plague, scaring away prospective recruits (ibid.: Feb. 24, 1911: 418). Without trained medical staff to assist them in their inspections, the Shenyang police often mistook those suffering from other diseases for plague victims. Those indiscriminately rounded up soon became infected and died in the quarantine stations (ibid.: Mar. 3, 1911: 488). Such treatment further undermined what little confidence the Shenyang population had in the plague prevention authorities. The number of police was also inadequate: the majority were assigned to inspection duty within the city, but this left too few sentries around its perimeter, so guards found it impossible to keep refugees fleeing the epidemic from fanning out into the countryside (ibid.: Feb. 24, 1911: 418).

Money was also quite limited. Xiliang, the governor-general of the Three Eastern Provinces, continually appealed to the central Ministry of Finance for funds with which to contain the epidemic (NCH Jan. 20, 1911: 154). As the epidemic spread, however, and as more appeals for money came in from other areas of the northeast, the Ministry of Finance requested imperial sanction to stop disbursements of funds. The Ministry claimed that its outlay already exceeded 10 million taels and that it no longer had the resources to meet the requests coming in from provincial authorities (ibid.: Mar. 10, 1911: 540).

Recognizing that the efforts of the official Plague Prevention Bureau were inadequate, local Han merchant-elite in the Shenyang Chamber of Commerce (Shangwu zonghui) stepped in and organized variants of Western-style public health agencies.[20] The local Chamber of Commerce set up its own "modern" health institutions, organizing both an isolation hospital for city merchants and its own plague inspection brigade.[21] Other corporate groups followed suit: for example, the small community of Muslims residing in Shenyang opened its own isolation ward (Shengjing shibao Feb. 18, 1911: 5).

The Plague Prevention Bureau initially approved of these nonofficial efforts, seeing them as an important auxiliary to the antiplague measures organized by the Shenyang police. Indeed, at the outset, it even helped organize the extrabureaucratic elite into a "temporary" Plague Prevention Association (*Linshi fangyi hui*; see Zhang Yuanqi 1911, 2: 14). The members of the association were drawn from the Shenyang Chamber of Commerce, the Shenyang Agricultural Association (*Nongwu hui*), and the Shenyang Self-Government Assembly (*Zizhi hui*; see *Shengjing shibao* Jan. 18, 1911: 5). Government reports on the epidemic make it clear that Chinese officials anticipated that the Plague Prevention Association would merely assist the police rather than supplant police-directed activities (Zhang Yuanqi 1911, 2: 14).

The directors of the Chamber of Commerce were careful to present their planned hospital as supplementary to official efforts (*Shengjing shibao* Jan. 17, 1911: 5, Feb. 11, 1911: 5). Publicly, they indicated that they were opening the isolation hospital because there were too few doctors, both Chinese and Western, to provide for all the merchants needing treatment in Shenyang. Privately, however, the Chamber appears to have been attempting to ameliorate some of the harsher aspects of Western-style quarantine for its own constituency. The merchant association was not opposed to Western medical techniques per se; indeed, it actively sought out Western-trained doctors to run the hospital, and only after its requests for a foreign physician were turned down by the Plague Prevention Bureau did the Chamber of Commerce hire two famous practitioners of Chinese medicine. Nor did the merchants reject the concept of isolation wards out of hand. The Chamber's clinic was partially designed as an infectious disease hospital along Western lines. Patients who were clearly infected with plague were kept on one side of the complex; all others were kept on another.

However, certain regulations were more relaxed in the Chamber hospital than they were in clinics run by the Plague Prevention Bureau. The merchants allowed family members to visit patients, and the Chinese doctors did not wear masks or use disinfectant before moving back and forth between the two wards. As a consequence, they inadvertently carried the infection from one side of the hospital to the other, and it was not long before everyone had become infected with the disease. Only a few weeks after the hospital opened, some two hundred fifty people had died, including both of the doctors (*NCH* Mar. 10, 1911: 554).

By establishing its own, less restrictive isolation hospital, the Chamber of Commerce seemed to be attempting to provide a form of care that would both be acceptable to its merchant constituency and incorporate the most essential elements of the Western model. Indeed, the

merchant community responded to these efforts as a compromise between Western and Chinese practice: merchants vigorously resisted
government efforts at plague control but voluntarily cooperated with
the measures initiated by the guilds. Instead of hiding their sick relatives at home, away from the eyes of the plague prevention authorities,
many brought them to the Chamber's hospital for treatment (NCH
Mar. 10, 1911: 554). Tragically, many previously uninfected persons
contracted plague and died while in the clinic.

When the high death rate in the merchants' hospital became known,
the provincial government ordered it closed on the grounds that it
was not using adequate sanitary or medical procedures.[22] The commissioner of foreign affairs also threatened to abolish the supplementary inspection brigade set up by the Chamber of Commerce and to
arrest any nonofficial person caught conducting plague inspections.[23]
Despite these threats, the Chamber's sanitary brigade continued its
work of cleaning up public wells, searching for victims and corpses in
the city's streets, and conducting house-to-house inspections. It was
only disbanded in April, after the epidemic had subsided.[24] The primary targets of these inspections were rickshaw pullers, prostitutes,
coolies, and beggars (Shengjing shibao Jan. 29, 1911: 5).

The Chamber of Commerce's involvement during the epidemic thus
went in two directions. On the one hand, the Shenyang elite, through
their establishment of a privately run plague isolation hospital, sought
to protect the merchant community from the more intrusive aspects of
the new police-directed disease control measures. On the other hand,
the Chamber of Commerce provided the authorities with an auxiliary
corps of inspectors, who actively participated in policing and surveillance activities.

That the nonofficial elite both cooperated and competed with the
authorities during the 1910–11 epidemic is not surprising. Shenyang
was primarily an administrative city and was situated in the home-
land of the ruling Manchus. Thus Han merchants did not have the
same political power there that their counterparts wielded in commercial cities to the south. Moreover, by 1911 there had been something of
a convergence in elite attitudes regarding Western-style public health.
The benefits of scientific medicine and the regulatory role of the modern state in protecting the public's health were increasingly accepted
by bureaucrats and nonofficial reformers alike. Although the Chamber of Commerce contested the extent to which merchants should be
subject to the new regulations, it also cooperated actively with the

police in monitoring the movement of other, more marginal members of society: laborers, transients, and the poor.

Conclusion

The seventeen years between 1894 and 1911 saw a transformation in the attitudes of some elite Chinese toward state medicine and Western-style public health. In 1894, when the British colonial authorities were forcefully introducing quarantine and isolation wards in Hong Kong, these measures met with both elite and popular resistance. The idea of state medicine began to take hold in China only after the Sino-Japanese War. Reform-minded intellectuals and some Qing officials began to call for the extension of Western-style public health institutions from Hong Kong and the treaty ports to the interior. In the political and ideological climate of the post-Boxer reform era, in which Western and Japanese institutional models were increasingly favored, there was a growing acceptance of the concept that the government was obliged to protect the public's health. By the time pneumonic plague broke out in Manchuria in 1910–11, new-style police in some Chinese municipalities were beginning to put this idea into practice.

The story of plague in Shenyang shows both similarities to and differences from the cases in Hong Kong and Canton discussed in Chapter 5. Whereas in 1894 Cantonese officials remained largely uninvolved in plague relief efforts, in 1911 key players in the Chinese-state administrative elite authorized the use of quarantine and detention of plague patients. The merchant-elite of Shenyang showed a limited accommodation to these governmental policies. Although the members of the Shenyang Chamber of Commerce accepted the necessity of stopping the plague, their effort to set up a plague hospital for merchants is reminiscent of the hospices established by Cantonese *shantang* and the Hong Kong–based Donghua Hospital. In 1894 Chinese civic activists attempted to mute the impact of colonial medicine; in 1911 the Shenyang elite tried to minimize the force of invasive Qing police actions.

State intervention during public health emergencies undeniably benefits society as a whole, and using the police as primary public-health officers remains a widespread and efficacious way to deal with highly lethal and contagious diseases. Indeed, the tragic outcome in the hospital set up by the Shenyang Chamber of Commerce suggests the consequences of nonintervention. While recognizing that state-sponsored public health is often a good and necessary thing, it should also be acknowledged that such policies brought people under state control in unprecedented ways. Hence the development of police-directed public health agencies in response to the threat of plague can be viewed as an important element in the history of early-twentieth-century Chinese state expansion.

After the Republican Revolution and the subsequent disintegration of central state control, there was a hiatus in state medical reform. Initiatives in public health devolved to regional institutions such as the North Manchurian Plague Prevention Service (Nathan 1967; Wu 1959). Truly effective public-health measures had to await greater political stability and the development of new state institutions later in the century (Lucas 1982). Nonetheless, the aspirations of Chinese state-builders were becoming clear in the New Policies period: civic activism in the realm of medical relief and public health was eventually to be curbed by an increasingly expansive state.

Conclusion

EPIDEMIC DISEASE in general, and plague in particular, was a familiar feature of the late imperial Chinese landscape. It was not only a biological but also a cultural phenomenon. From its origins in eighteenth-century Yunnan to its explosion on the world scene as the third pandemic in the late nineteenth century, plague followed the paths of Chinese trade, reflected changes in China's regional systems, and was part of the massive political and social dislocations that characterized the waning days of the Qing.

As an unpredictable and uncontrollable act of fate, plague seemed to be a sign of the gods' displeasure or of the anguish of wandering ghosts. Individual people, local elite, and Qing officials alike sought celestial intervention; they also did what they could to ease the pain of plague victims. As Western influence began to penetrate the Chinese continent, it, too, became an integral part of the history of plague. Colonial efforts at plague control provoked both resistance and reform, eventually leading to plague eradication campaigns modeled on Western- and Japanese-style public health measures. The supervision and regulation of health and sanitation, begun by foreigners in Hong Kong and in the treaty ports, were ultimately assumed by a modernizing Chinese state with aspirations toward greater control over local society.

The story of plague in Qing China is thus intertwined with a number of themes central to late imperial Chinese history. The appearance of plague in Yunnan and its spread to the southeastern littoral were directly connected with movements of populations and goods that reflected frontier expansion over the course of the Qing period. Foreign interventions during plague outbreaks link this story to the political impact of imperialism on China and the ways in which European cultural representations of the Chinese influenced the theory and practice of colonial medicine. Finally, the police-directed public health initiatives of the New Policies reform era are an example of new forms of state-societal interaction that emerged in the last decade of Qing rule.

In the eyes of many nineteenth-century Europeans and Americans, plague marked China as a hygienically "backward" country that continued to incubate a medieval disease in the modern era. For them, plague was yet another indication of the deterioration of the so-called Sick Man of Asia. Western doctors explained plague's origins in Yunnan by noting that the disease had appeared concurrently with the Muslim Rebellion of 1856–73, a conflict "conspicuous for so many massacres and attended by so many miseries" (Inspectorate General, *Customs Medical Reports* 1894, No. 48: 41). Reports that plague had appeared earlier in Yunnan, during the height of eighteenth-century prosperity, were dismissed as "incompatible with the conditions of misery necessary to the development of such an infectious germ as that of *yang-tzu-ping* [*yangzibing*]" (ibid.; see also Simpson 1905: 50).

The Qing epidemics also solidified the European view that China was the "original home of plague" and the source of the European Black Death (Wu 1936: 11). As John Norris (1977: 5) has observed, nineteenth-century European prejudice, self-confidence, and perceptions of "technologically primitive" nations created a readiness to accept such a view. Perversely, this view was actually strengthened by the development of the germ theory, "even though, by 1914, it had been determined that plague was not a 'filth' disease. The fact that the third pandemic originated from Southwestern China seemed to clinch the matter: if plague originated in China in the nineteenth century, why not in the fourteenth as well?" (ibid.).

Although the ultimate source of the Black Death remains obscure, it seems indisputable that China was the point of origin for the modern pandemic, given the chronology of plague outbreaks around the world at the turn of the century. However, the reasons plague began in Yunnan and spread throughout much of southern China were quite different from those portrayed in early studies. While it is true that the Muslim Rebellion and its "attendant miseries" led to widespread outbreaks of plague in the 1860's and 1870's, the disease was already present in Yunnan during the more prosperous eighteenth century. Initially it was not a sign of decay at all, but of economic vigor and vitality. Plague appeared in human communities after an expanding population intruded into the natural habitats of plague-carrying animals, and it became more than a local issue because remote areas were linked to other regions by systems of long-distance transport. When Han immigrants moved into Yunnan in the mid-eighteenth century, they opened up new land, increased trade, and formed new commercial networks. These transformations provided the preconditions for the spread of plague to human settlements, which can thus be seen as an undesirable side effect of economic development in a region where plague was already enzootic.

The diffusion of plague outside of Yunnan was also associated with an increase in economic activity. In the eighteenth century, the distance separating the southwest from the rest of the empire was simply too great to allow for much interregional commerce. Yet in the first half of the nineteenth century, trade in domestic opium stimulated greater movement between Yunnan and the Lingnan region. As a result, Yunnan became part of a larger market economy. In the 1850's social disorder and civil strife diverted the Yunnan-Lingnan opium traffic through Beihai and the Leizhou Peninsula, an area that supports the main plague-carrier in southern China, the yellow-chested rat. This combination of human agency (changes in routes used to transport domestically grown opium) and the interaction of humans with the natural environment (movement through the habitats of rodents capable of carrying and transmitting plague) allowed bubonic plague to spread eventually throughout much of southern China.

A similar process of economic expansion into the periphery, albeit over a much shorter period of time, gave rise to the 1910–11 pneumonic plague epidemic in Manchuria. Until the early twentieth century, isolated pockets of enzootic plague in Mongolia and Siberia remained largely undisturbed. Railroad construction, the market demands of the international fur trade, and the loosening of controls over Han immigration into Manchuria stimulated the large-scale movement of fur trappers into these wilderness areas. Once pneumonic plague broke out among migrants, the newly constructed Manchurian railway system allowed for rapid plague diffusion throughout the entire northeast. Again, plague was largely a consequence of incursions into a wilderness area combined with new linkages between the periphery and the regional core. It was not accidental that plague erupted in China during two centuries of unprecedented population growth and economic expansion along the frontier.

In many ways, the image of a decaying China presented in earlier analyses of the late Qing epidemics reflects nineteenth-century Western preconceptions and prejudices about China and the Chinese. During an era of intensive imperialist expansion and unshaken belief in the superiority of Western science, Europeans and North Americans used scientific and technological achievement as a measure of civilization (Adas 1989: 194). For many, China was a "barbaric" and "semi-civilized" country that had advanced early on but had then stagnated and declined. As their comments during the plague epidemics indicate, nineteenth-century colonial physicians, administrators, and missionaries viewed Chinese responses to plague from this vantage point. They condemned Chinese officials for their supposed indifference to the plight of victims and ridiculed the masses for their "superstitious" religious festivals and processionals.

Foreigners conceived of Western medicine and public health as a necessary corrective for the "benighted" Chinese, whom they assumed were ignorant of even the most basic principles of sanitation. Any antipathy to these measures on the part of the Chinese was imagined to be motivated by conservative opposition to modern scientific knowledge. Thus, in European narratives of the 1894 plague epidemic in Hong Kong, the resistance of the Chinese community to British plague policies was interpreted as a "rigid" adherence to "tradition" and a reluctance to embrace "progress." This was contrasted with the heroic efforts of a colonial government striving to bring modern science and public health to a regressive nation.

Contrary to these late-nineteenth-century perspectives, which are tethered to what Paul Cohen (1984) has termed the "tradition-modernity" and "impact-response" modes of explanation, this study has sought to provide a more nuanced and balanced account of the introduction of Western public-health institutions into China. At the turn of the century, as in the present, both Chinese and Western medicine were continuing to evolve. Discussions between Warm Factor and Cold Damage theorists indicate that late-Qing medical theory and practice was the subject of ongoing debate. Nor was biomedicine fully formed at the time. Indeed, epidemiology, microbiology, and tropical medicine were all relatively new fields of investigation in the 1880's and 1890's. Viewed from this perspective, British colonial interventions during the 1894 Hong Kong epidemic were not exclusively rational, efficacious responses to an emergency medical situation, nor were the Chinese reactions to these policies merely irrational rejections of a transparently superior medical system. Rather, actions and attitudes on both sides were the product of the complex interplay between pre-existing cultural systems of meaning and historically specific circumstances.

The antiplague measures undertaken by the Hong Kong government in 1894 were not based on a complete knowledge of plague epidemiology, nor did they lead invariably to effective interventions. A number of factors shaped policy: the emerging microbiological revolution, the nineteenth-century state medical movement, as well as preconceptions about Chinese society and the wider orientalist discourse within which nineteenth-century "tropical" medicine was embedded (Anderson 1992: 506–29). Tropical medicine was initially based on a belief that European constitutions were endangered not only by warm climates but also by the imagined "lack of hygiene" of colonial subjects. Indigenous populations were seen as the source of contagion and as part of a dangerous environment that had to be controlled and contained.

These ideas influenced European views of plague etiology. Despite the identification of plague's causal agent in 1894, its mode of transmission remained a mystery to most Western physicians and scientists for many years after the third pandemic began. Modern plague-control measures—such as rat-proofing buildings and transport vehicles, catching and poisoning rats, and using insecticides to destroy rat fleas—were all twentieth-century developments that were unavailable to Hong Kong authorities at the turn of the century. Many Western doctors working in China at the time remained convinced that plague was a "filth" disease caused by the "uncivilized" living conditions of the Chinese. These images precipitated colonial policy along three intrusive, but not uniformly effective, lines: a massive cleanup campaign of the poorest Chinese neighborhoods (generally by burning down houses); the isolation of plague patients from their families; and an effort to prevent Chinese residents both from entering European enclaves and from leaving the colony. Not surprisingly, these policies provoked resistance on the part of the Chinese community. In the face of this opposition, the Hong Kong government was unable to enforce a strict sanitation blockade, one measure that might have stemmed the further spread of the disease.

Nor were Chinese responses to these interventions merely unthinking rejections of scientific medicine. While there was clearly much in European clinical practice that was alien to Chinese experience, many Chinese appear to have accepted Western medicine when it was provided in ways that were familiar—such as drug therapy—and when it was proven to be effective. Opposition in Hong Kong centered on those policies—quarantine, the destruction of property, and the use of isolation wards—which implied a loss of personal control. Not only did hospitalization mean removal from one's own residence, it also did not ensure survival, given the 90 percent case-fatality rates recorded in foreign clinics. Chinese residents' protests against the interference of the colonial state in their lives thus reflected both deeply held cultural values and "situated and highly articulate practical responses to specific historical pressures" as well (Farquhar and Hevia 1993: 507).

Resistance to British colonial medicine in Hong Kong was led by elite activists working through post-Taiping philanthropic organizations such as the Donghua Hospital and the *Aiyu shantang*. This was not simply conservative obstructionism, however, because these corporations also responded aggressively to the crisis posed by plague, providing a wide array of assistance that ranged from free medical care to charitable burials. Similar civic efforts had been the norm in England and the United States only a few decades before, but by the turn of the century, public health was increasingly viewed as an important function of the modern state. Foreign commentators condemned the Chinese civic response as yet another sign of China's weakness. European governments, sharing the same views and troubled by the continued global diffusion of plague, brought increasing pressure on the Qing court to adopt strict quarantine rules, travel restrictions, and other policies considered essential to arresting its spread.

By the end of the century, some of these same issues began to be raised by Chinese reformers, both in and out of the government. Figures as prominent as Kang Youwei appealed for the establishment of "modern" and "progressive" state medical institutions. Faced with these internal calls for sanitation reform and worried that the lack of a centralized public-health bureaucracy would provide the foreign powers with an excuse to intervene further, concerned Qing officials eventually moved to institute Western- and Japanese-style public health measures. Beginning in 1902, activist officials such as Cen

Chunxuan, Zhao Erxun, and Yuan Shikai established modern police-directed public health bureaus in a number of provinces, including Sichuan, Zhili, and Fengtian. In the fall of 1910 and the winter of 1911, when plague broke out in Manchuria, epidemic control measures were directed largely by such new-style police.

Late-nineteenth-century Chinese reactions to plague and to Western ideas about its treatment and control are thus part of a broader set of questions about the interaction of the Chinese state and society in the late Qing period. Between 1894, when plague appeared in Hong Kong and Canton, and 1911, when it spread throughout the northeast, two visions of the state-society relationship were increasingly coming into conflict. On the one hand, activist elite, such as the Donghua Directorate and members of the Shenyang Chamber of Commerce, desired greater involvement in local government. Their philanthropic activities during plague epidemics, like their public management of schools, local militias, and water control, can be seen as a manifestation of this reach for greater self-government. On the other hand, Qing officials recognized the need to build a fiscally and militarily strong state in the face of substantial foreign threats, and therefore initiated a number of measures designed to recover imperial state control over society. This state-building effort extended into societal spheres as diverse as taxation, the suppression of popular religion, the building of "model" prisons, and the incarceration of mental patients (Diamant 1992; Duara 1988a: 58–85; Duara 1991: 67–83; Dutton 1992: 157–78). The development of police-directed public health agencies was consistent with this more general trend toward state penetration of local society.

As this study has attempted to demonstrate, the social history of disease is not only a significant subject in its own right but can also reveal important aspects of Chinese economic, political, social, and cultural life in the last century of Qing rule. The patterns in which plague spread, the ways in which people tried to control the disease, and the manner in which they interpreted their suffering have allowed this investigation of plague in Qing China to document not simply the story of how the Chinese died, but also how they lived.

APPENDIXES

Patterns of Plague Morbidity and Mortality in Taiwan, 1897-1917, and Hong Kong, 1893-1923

PLAGUE'S DEMOGRAPHIC impact can be assessed only by using relative measures based on reliable cause-of-death statistics and accurate population data. Regrettably, for most of the Chinese communities affected by the disease in the Qing period, such data simply do not exist. The only comprehensive measures of plague morbidity and mortality in nineteenth- and early-twentieth-century China come from two areas under the control of foreign governments. Beginning in the mid-1890's, both the British government in Hong Kong and the Japanese government on Taiwan collected statistics on plague in their respective colonies. Some of these data were presented in Chapter 5; these appendixes provide further information on plague morbidity and mortality in Hong Kong and Taiwan.

Although the available statistics on plague morbidity and mortality add to our understanding of the impact of plague on Taiwan and in Hong Kong, they cannot shed much light on the effects of plague in China proper because conditions in these two colonies were not representative of those elsewhere. In the 1890's Western plague-control measures were generally ineffective, but in the first decade of the twentieth century both the British and the Japanese began implementing measures (such as ship quarantine and rat-catching) that may have served to lessen infection (and hence mortality). No such preventive policies were in effect in Qing China before 1911. Thus, while morbidity and mortality rates on the mainland were probably the same as or higher than those recorded for Taiwan and Hong Kong, it is not possible to verify this presumption statistically.

Plague Morbidity and Mortality in Hong Kong, 1894-1923, and Taiwan, 1897-1917

TABLES A.1 AND A.2 show the number of recorded plague cases and deaths and relative plague morbidity and mortality rates in Hong Kong from 1894 through 1923 and in Taiwan from 1897 through 1917. For both colonies, plague-specific death rates per thousand residents were considerably lower than those recorded in or estimated for other areas of the world. Between 1894 and 1923, the annual plague-mortality rate in Hong Kong never exceeded 11 persons per thousand, and for most years it was considerably below that. Plague death rates in Taiwan were even lower; during the worst outbreak, in 1901, there were only 1.3 plague deaths per thousand residents. In contrast, for some areas of twentieth-century India, mortality rates of 100 per thousand are on record (Klein 1988: 724). Plague mortality in Hong Kong and Taiwan did not compare even to the relatively low levels documented in Indonesia. After plague reached Java in 1910, a few districts had plague deaths above 20 per thousand (Hull 1987: note 6).

These comparisons are somewhat misleading, at least in the case of Taiwan, because they contrast disaggregated data from India and Java to aggregated Taiwan data. Plague seldom affects an entire region all at once, and using provincial or national population figures has the effect of lowering the death rate. When national census data were used to calculate plague mortality for twentieth-century India, for example, the results were extremely low (from 0.20 to 5 per 1,000). The very high rate of 100 per thousand just noted was recorded only after statistics were divided into smaller geographical units (Klein 1988: 724).

TABLE A.1

Plague Morbidity and Mortality in Hong Kong, 1894–1923

Year	Population (mid-year)	Plague cases	Plague deaths	Plague cases per 1,000	Plague deaths per 1,000	Case-fatality rate
1894	242,365	2,679	2,552	11.05	10.53	95.26%
1895	247,252	45	36	0.18	0.15	80.00
1896	243,959	1,204	1,078	4.94	4.42	89.53
1897	244,065	21	19	0.09	0.08	90.48
1898	251,555	1,320	1,175	5.25	4.67	89.02
1899	256,856	1,486	1,434	5.79	5.58	96.50
1900	260,995	1,057	1,022	4.05	3.92	96.69
1901	281,669	1,651	1,562	5.86	5.55	94.61
1902	306,242	572	559	1.87	1.83	97.73
1903	318,728	1,415	1,249	4.44	3.92	88.27
1904	343,419	510	493	1.49	1.44	96.67
1905	369,528	304	287	0.82	0.78	94.41
1906	329,038	893	842	2.71	2.56	94.29
1907	329,198	240	198	0.73	0.60	82.50
1908	375,428	1,073	986	2.86	2.63	91.89
1909	425,194	135	108	0.32	0.25	80.00
1910	432,437	25	23	0.06	0.05	92.00
1911	450,132	269	253	0.60	0.56	94.05
1912	466,027	1,847	1,768	3.96	3.79	95.72
1913	478,446	408	386	0.85	0.81	94.61
1914	495,209	2,146	2,020	4.33	4.08	94.13
1915	505,232	144	144	0.29	0.29	100.00
1916	518,585	39	38	0.08	0.07	97.44
1917	531,555	38	38	0.07	0.07	100.00
1918	548,300	266	266	0.49	0.49	100.00
1919	579,800	464	464	0.80	0.80	100.00
1920	614,204	138	120	0.22	0.20	86.96
1921	627,737	150	130	0.24	0.21	86.67
1922	631,733	1,181	1,071	1.87	1.70	90.69
1923	653,100	148	136	0.23	0.21	91.89

SOURCE: Hong Kong Government 1932, *Historical and Statistical Abstracts,* and ibid.. 1894–1908, *Hong Kong Legislative Council Sessional Papers.*

NOTE: 1897, 1901, 1911, and 1921 were census years.

Table A.3 provides an example of how mortality rates differ spatially when disaggregated data are available. Between 1898 and 1907, plague-specific death rates in Taiwan were very low when the island's entire population was used. As noted in Table A.1, for 1901, the worst plague year on record, only 1.3 plague deaths per thousand were recorded for the island as a whole. Yet during the same year, Tainan subprefecture (*ting*) had a plague-specific death rate of 6 per thousand, while Taibei and Jiayi subprefectures each had a rate of 4 per thou-

TABLE A.2

Plague Morbidity and Mortality in Taiwan, 1897–1917

Year	Population[a] (mid-year)	Plague cases	Plague deaths	Plague cases per 1,000	Plague deaths per 1,000	Case-fatality rate
1897	2,715,443	730	566	0.27	0.21	77.53%
1898	2,613,433	1,233	882	0.47	0.34	71.53
1899	2,658,829	2,637	1,995	0.99	0.75	75.65
1900	2,745,276	1,079	809	0.39	0.29	74.98
1901	2,830,749	4,496	3,670	1.59	1.30	81.63
1902	2,902,146	2,308	1,969	0.80	0.68	85.31
1903	2,922,585	885	708	0.30	0.24	80.00
1904	2,969,349	4,494	3,370	1.51	1.13	74.99
1905	3,038,636	2,388	2,090	0.79	0.69	87.52
1906	3,070,254	3,267	2,604	1.06	0.85	79.71
1907	3,097,327	2,586	2,235	0.83	0.72	86.43
1908	3,120,184	1,270	1,059	0.41	0.34	83.39
1909	3,154,613	1,026	848	0.33	0.27	82.65
1910	3,204,271	19	18	0.01	0.01	94.74
1911	3,272,573	378	332	0.12	0.10	87.83
1912	3,336,014	223	185	0.07	0.06	82.96
1913	3,399,106	136	125	0.04	0.04	91.91
1914	3,449,137	566	487	0.16	0.14	86.04
1915	3,465,041	74	66	0.02	0.02	89.19
1916	3,491,487	5	4	0.00	0.00	80.00
1917	3,540,837	7	7	0.00	0.00	100.00

SOURCE: Government-General of Taiwan (Taiwan Sōtokufu) 1924:7–8.
[a]Taiwanese and Japanese population only; aboriginal population not included.

sand. In 1899 islandwide plague mortality was only 0.75 per thousand (see Table A.2), but in Tainan the rate was nearly 9 per thousand. To be sure, even these disaggregated figures are very low relative to the Indian experience. Nonetheless, they give some sense of the spatial differentiation in plague mortality we would expect to see if similar records existed for other areas of China.

TABLE A.3

Plague-Specific Death Rates per Thousand for Twenty Subprefectures of Taiwan, 1897–1917

Location	1897	1898	1899	1900	1901	1902	1903	1904	1905	1906	1907	1908	1909	1910	1911	1912	1913	1914	1915	1916	1917
Taibei	0.08	0.50	0.76	1.10	4.16	3.19	1.25	1.42	2.11	1.64	3.61	—	—	—	—	—	—	0.02	—	0.01	0.01
Jilong	0.05	0.07	0.04	0.03	0.31	0.51	0.34	0.20	0.20	0.04	0.87	—	—	—	—	—	—	—	—	—	—
Shenkeng	0.77	0.88	0.67	0.69	3.18	1.29	0.31	0.11	—	0.21	—	—	—	—	—	—	—	—	—	—	—
Yilan	—	—	—	—	0.01	—	—	—	2.74	—	—	—	—	—	—	—	—	—	—	—	—
Taoyuan	0.11	0.01	0.01	0.35	0.56	0.88	0.01	0.01	—	0.00	0.00	—	—	—	—	—	—	—	—	—	—
Xinzhu	0.07	0.40	0.13	0.05	0.02	0.18	0.74	0.21	2.38	—	0.02	—	—	—	—	—	—	—	—	—	—
Miaoli	—	—	—	0.01	—	0.01	—	—	0.01	0.22	—	—	—	—	—	—	—	—	—	—	—
Taizhong	—	0.14	0.01	0.03	0.29	—	—	—	—	—	—	0.34	—	—	—	—	—	—	—	—	—
Zhanghua	0.22	1.88	0.07	0.01	—	—	—	—	—	0.03	0.04	—	—	—	—	—	—	—	—	—	—
Nantou	—	—	0.31	0.59	0.04	—	—	—	—	—	—	—	—	—	—	—	—	—	—	—	—
Douliu	0.01	0.66	—	0.02	0.04	0.05	—	0.17	0.02	0.67	—	0.31	—	—	—	—	—	—	—	—	—
Jiayi	—	—	—	0.20	4.00	0.16	0.62	4.17	2.09	4.04	2.39	2.46	0.85	0.02	0.62	0.34	0.22	0.85	0.12	—	—
Yanshuigang	—	—	0.19	0.84	0.61	1.02	0.18	2.38	0.73	0.81	0.86	0.55	—	—	—	—	—	—	—	—	—
Tainan	2.47	0.35	8.93	0.58	6.44	0.80	0.10	7.86	0.64	1.17	0.44	0.76	0.08	0.01	—	—	—	—	—	—	—
Fengshan	—	—	0.86	0.02	1.05	1.16	—	0.04	0.01	3.77	1.12	0.55	—	—	—	—	—	—	—	—	—
Fanshucai	—	—	0.99	0.16	0.02	0.04	—	—	—	—	—	—	—	—	—	—	—	—	—	—	—
Agou	—	—	—	0.08	0.01	0.01	—	—	—	0.03	0.16	—	—	—	—	—	—	—	—	—	—
Hengchun	—	—	—	—	—	—	—	—	—	—	—	—	—	—	—	—	—	—	—	—	—
Taidong	—	—	—	—	—	—	—	—	—	—	—	—	—	—	—	—	—	—	—	—	—
Penghu	—	—	0.02	—	—	—	—	—	—	—	—	0.77	—	—	—	—	—	—	—	—	—
All island	0.21	0.34	0.75	0.30	1.30	0.64	0.24	1.14	0.69	0.83	0.72	0.34	0.27	0.006	0.10	0.06	0.04	0.14	0.02	0.00	0.00

SOURCES: Provincial Government of Taiwan, Bureau of Accounting and Statistics, 1946: 80–81; *Taiwan sheng tongzhigao* 1951–60, vol. 3, part 7b: 72–74.

Comparative Causes of Death in Hong Kong, 1893-1907, and Taiwan, 1897-1906

IN ADDITION TO cause-specific death rates, epidemiologists use a measure known as the proportionate mortality ratio (PMR) to assess the relative importance of a particular cause of death in relation to all deaths in a population. This ratio (derived by dividing the number of deaths from a given cause in a specified time period by the total deaths in the same period) is useful in assessing the proportion of lives lost due to a particular cause of death. When measuring PMRs over a period of time, it is important to take into account not only the average ratio but also the coefficient of variability (derived by dividing the standard deviation by the average). This coefficient enables us to distinguish endemic diseases, which represent a constant but stable threat, from epidemic diseases, which generally vary greatly from year to year. Endemic diseases typically have a low coefficient of variability; the coefficient of variability for epidemic diseases is usually somewhat higher.

As indicated in Table B.1, plague was one of the leading causes of death in Hong Kong throughout the first decade of the twentieth century. Between 1893 and 1907, plague represented, on average, 12.57 percent of all causes of death in the colony, and it killed 307 people for every 100,000 residents (or 3 per 1,000). According to recorded statistics, as shown in Table B.2, it was the major single cause of death by disease, surpassing pulmonary tuberculosis (average annual PMR = 9.92 percent) and malaria (7.49 percent). Tuberculosis and malaria had lower coefficients of variability than did plague (testifying to their con-

Causes of Death in Hong Kong, 1893–1907

Cause of death	Total deaths by cause, 1893–1907	Average annual proportional mortality ratio (PMR), 1893–1907	Coeff. of varia- bility	Average annual cause- specific death rate per 100,000, 1893–1907	Coeff. of varia- bility
Class I. General Diseases					
A. Febrile disease					
1. Zymotic diseases					
Plague	12,506	12.57	0.82	306.69	0.94
Smallpox	1,078	1.15	1.14	25.15	1.08
Measles	39	0.04	1.35	0.96	1.42
Typhoid/typhus	1,603	1.74	1.41	42.48	1.48
Continued fevers	126	0.16	2.36	3.20	2.23
Cholera	617	0.62	2.75	13.57	2.77
Dysentery	1,390	1.45	0.46	32.90	0.47
Diphtheria	68	0.07	1.25	1.51	1.24
Whooping cough	15	0.02	1.93	0.35	2.04
Influenza	10	0.01	1.08	0.23	1.12
Dengue fever	5	0.005	2.19	0.10	2.14
Diarrhea (infant)	3,171	3.17	0.76	71.56	0.80
Chicken pox	3	0.003	2.07	0.07	2.10
Scarlet fever	2	0.002	2.68	0.04	2.64
Mumps	1	0.001	3.87	0.03	3.87
Cerebrospinal fever	1	0.001	3.87	0.02	3.87
2. Malaria	6,977	7.49	0.35	169.95	0.35
3. Septicaemia	526	0.54	0.49	12.03	0.52
4. Venereal disease					
Syphilis	707	0.70	0.75	15.67	0.80
5. Zoogenous disease					
Rabies	3	0.003	2.08	0.08	2.07
B. Deaths due to external agents					
1. Parasites	55	0.06	1.23	1.45	1.43
2. Injuries/poisoning	3,443	3.44	0.57	78.81	0.65
C. Developmental disorders					
Old age, premature births, etc.	9,344	9.64	0.37	211.38	0.31
D. Miscellaneous diseases					
Cancer and other	2,855	2.81	0.87	60.34	0.85
Beriberi	5,118	5.21	0.61	112.45	0.52
Class II. Local Diseases					
A. Diseases of the respiratory system					
Pulmonary tuberculosis	9,392	9.92	0.33	220.93	0.35
Bronchitis	6,037	6.48	0.25	145.41	0.23
Pneumonia	4,483	4.49	0.73	102.31	0.77
Other	774	0.81	0.45	17.95	0.42
B. Diseases of the nervous system					

TABLE B.1 *(continued)*

Cause of death	Total deaths by cause, 1893–1907	Average annual proportional mortality ratio (PMR), 1893–1907	Coeff. of varia- bility	Average annual cause- specific death rate per 100,000, 1893–1907	Coeff. of varia- bility
Class II. Local Diseases					
(continued)					
Tetanus/trismus	7,293	7.90	0.51	183.09	0.56
Infant convulsions	3,529	3.91	0.66	90.99	0.68
Cerebrospinal meningitis	1,275	1.25	1.02	26.77	1.03
Other	1,059	1.13	0.32	25.47	0.35
C. *Diseases of the digestive system (not including diarrhea)*	2,961	3.28	0.82	75.52	0.85
D. *Diseases of the circulatory system*	2,035	2.12	0.34	46.82	0.31
E. *Diseases of the urinary tract*	797	0.85	0.39	18.94	0.41
F. *Reproductive system disorders (not including venereal disease)*	45	0.05	0.89	1.17	0.88
G. *Skin disease*	212	0.23	1.83	5.35	1.84
H. *Diseases of limbs (gangrene)*	88	0.10	0.90	2.25	0.93
I. *Pregnancy and childbirth*	562	0.59	0.32	13.65	0.39
Class III. Ill-defined or Undiagnosed	5,627	6.02	0.55	137.07	0.59
ALL CAUSES OF DEATH	95,832	100.00	0.00	2,274.72	0.15

SOURCE: Hong Kong Government 1894–1908. *Hong Kong Legislative Council Sessional Papers.*
NOTE: These categories represent those used by the Hong Kong Government between 1893 and 1907. They do not necessarily correlate to biomedical terminology in use in the late twentieth century.

stant presence among the Hong Kong population), but plague itself varied less relative to its average than did other epidemic diseases such as cholera, typhoid, and smallpox.

These cause-of-death statistics probably do not reveal the entire picture of how Hong Kong residents died. Hong Kong sojourners, like Chinese sojourners elsewhere, tended to return home when they were ill. Those with diseases that killed slowly, such as malaria or tuberculosis, had ample time to leave the colony. In contrast, those who contracted plague often immediately became too ill to travel and, after only a few days, died in Hong Kong. Moreover, because Hong Kong's population was composed mostly of adult males, the proportions of

TABLE B.2
Proportionate Mortality Ratios (PMR) for Selected Diseases in Hong Kong, 1893–1907

Year	Plague	Malaria	Pulmonary tuberculosis	Cholera	Dysentery	Smallpox	Typhoid/ typhus	Diphtheria
1893	0.00	6.58	3.38	0.06	2.14	0.94	8.37	0.04
1894	34.45	4.16	1.69	0.09	1.24	0.24	5.95	0.00
1895	0.67	12.59	11.24	0.35	2.02	0.15	3.98	0.00
1896	18.40	9.10	10.67	0.38	1.47	0.20	2.37	0.03
1897	0.41	11.82	13.99	0.02	2.11	4.46	0.23	0.00
1898	20.71	9.34	12.43	0.05	1.15	1.94	0.41	0.07
1899	23.20	8.83	11.83	0.00	0.65	0.57	0.57	0.06
1900	15.09	8.19	12.89	0.01	0.89	0.25	0.80	0.12
1901	22.06	8.11	10.48	0.17	0.76	0.83	0.48	0.03
1902	8.24	6.27	10.92	6.71	1.37	0.60	0.35	0.07
1903	20.19	4.85	10.25	0.11	1.02	0.50	0.27	0.06
1904	8.06	4.92	9.14	0.69	0.56	0.65	1.03	0.03
1905	4.35	4.35	10.99	0.14	1.30	0.47	0.73	0.02
1906	10.05	5.35	9.75	0.02	2.48	1.68	0.24	0.12
1907	2.72	7.95	9.18	0.47	2.54	3.77	0.34	0.33
Average:	12.57	7.49	9.92	0.62	1.45	1.15	1.74	0.07
Std. deviation:	10.37	2.61	3.29	1.70	0.66	1.31	2.46	0.08
Coeff. of variability:	0.82	0.35	0.33	2.75	0.46	1.14	1.41	1.25

SOURCE: Hong Kong Government 1894–1908, *Hong Kong Legislative Council Sessional Papers*.

TABLE B.3
Proportionate Mortality Ratios (PMR) for Selected Diseases in Taiwan, 1898–1906

Year	Malaria	Plague	Cholera	Dysentery	Smallpox	Typhoid/typhus	Diphtheria
1898		4.38	0.00	0.13	0.17	0.09	0.01
1899	17.69	7.14	0.00	0.19	0.02	0.02	0.00
1900	15.15	1.60	0.00	0.05	0.03	0.01	0.00
1901	15.91	6.16	0.00	0.07	0.02	0.02	0.01
1902	17.59	2.48	0.64	0.20	0.01	0.02	0.00
1903	16.41	0.84	0.00	0.03	0.00	0.03	0.00
1904	12.45	3.54	0.00	0.03	0.00	0.02	0.01
1905	10.20	2.25	0.00	0.01	0.00	0.01	0.01
1906	10.00	2.50	0.00	0.03	0.00	0.03	0.01
Average:	14.43	3.65	0.06	0.12	0.06	0.03	0.01
Std. deviation:	3.13	2.10	0.20	0.13	0.12	0.02	0.00
Coeff. of variability:	0.22	0.58	3.16	1.12	1.92	0.94	0.53

SOURCES: Malaria data from Chen Shaoxing 1985 [1979]: 88–89; all others from Government-General of Taiwan (Taiwan Sōtokufu) 1924: 6–9.

NOTE: Taiwanese population only; Japanese and aboriginal population not included.

TABLE B.4
Causes of Death in Taiwan, 1906–15

Cause of death	Total deaths by cause, 1906–15	Average annual proportional mortality ratio (PMR), 1906–15	Coeff. of varia-bility	Average annual cause-specific death rate per 100,000, 1906–15	Coeff. of varia-bility
Class I. General Diseases					
A. Infectious/parasitic					
Malaria	94,741	9.87	0.15	294.25	0.24
Pulmonary tuberculosis	39,648	4.19	0.05	122.81	0.07
Other forms of tuberculosis	23,033	2.44	0.16	71.71	0.19
Plague	7,974	0.80	1.11	25.46	1.18
Influenza	4,522	0.48	0.23	14.03	0.27
Parasitic diseases	5,806	0.61	0.31	17.82	0.29
Measles	3,873	0.40	0.62	12.11	0.70
Dysentery	983	0.10	0.39	3.06	0.39
Whooping cough	1,307	0.14	0.33	4.05	0.31
Smallpox	179	0.02	0.67	0.55	0.72
Typhoid/typhus	237	0.03	0.30	0.73	0.27
Scarlet fever	15	0.00	1.19	0.05	1.25
Diphtheria	470	0.05	0.34	1.45	0.29
Syphilis	0	0.00	0.00	0.00	0.00
B. Other general diseases					
Diabetes	0	0.00	0.00	0.00	0.00
Cancer	7,141	0.72	0.96	22.64	1.00
Vitamin deficiencies (beriberi)	6,117	0.65	0.30	19.01	0.35
Class II. Local Diseases					
A. Diseases of the nervous system					
Meningitis	17,971	1.91	0.38	54.96	0.37
Cerebral hemorrhage/ stroke	13,734	1.45	0.07	42.69	0.16
Other nervous system diseases	4,489	0.48	0.13	13.89	0.10
B. Diseases of the circulatory system					
Heart disease	6,023	0.67	0.23	18.22	0.22
Other circulatory system diseases	4,146	0.41	0.54	13.32	0.48
C. Diseases of the respiratory system					
Bronchitis	39,314	4.19	0.33	120.62	0.31
Pneumonia	42,110	4.47	0.43	128.59	0.42
Other respiratory ailments (not including tuberculosis)	62,694	6.64	0.12	194.07	0.11

TABLE B.4 *(continued)*

Cause of death	Total deaths by cause, 1906–15	Average annual proportional mortality ratio (PMR), 1906–15	Coeff. of varia- bility	Average annual cause- specific death rate per 100,000, 1906–15	Coeff. of varia- bility
Class II. Local Diseases					
(continued)					
D. Diseases of the digestive system					
Stomach and intestinal ulcers	60,049	6.37	0.19	185.45	0.18
Diarrhea (infant and other)	75,340	8.03	0.29	231.28	0.24
Hernia	508	0.05	0.53	1.55	0.52
Cirrhosis of the liver	1,294	0.14	0.35	3.98	0.33
Other digestive system disorders	12,651	1.38	0.31	37.99	0.41
E. Diseases of the urinary tract	11,169	1.19	0.46	34.06	0.45
F. Diseases of the reproductive system	2,655	0.28	0.17	8.23	0.16
G. Childbirth and pregnancy	83,043	8.75	0.13	258.74	0.21
H. Skin and skeletal disease	0	0.00	0.00	0.00	0.00
I. Developmental disorders					
Congenital disorders	27,524	2.95	0.38	84.25	0.34
Old age	35,201	3.73	0.13	109.07	0.13
J. External injury					
Suicide	5,692	0.61	0.17	17.57	0.08
Accidental injury	16,068	1.68	0.32	49.70	0.38
Class III. Ill-defined or Undiagnosed	231,684	24.13	0.35	726.14	0.44
ALL CAUSES OF DEATH	949,405	100.00	0.00	2,944.07	0.11

SOURCE: Provincial Government of Taiwan, Bureau of Accounting and Statistics 1946: 269–77.
NOTE: These categories represent those used by the Japanese colonial government in Taiwan between 1906 and 1915. They do not necessarily correlate to biomedical terminology in use in the late twentieth century.

deaths due to natural causes in old age, infant diarrhea, and during pregnancy and childbirth were quite low.

Plague was an important cause of death in Taiwan as well. During the period (1897–1906) when plague was most prevalent on the island, comparative cause-of-death statistics are available only for malaria and for those diseases (plague, cholera, dysentery, smallpox, typhoid/typhus, and diphtheria) deemed legally notifiable by the Japanese authorities (Table B.3). Among these seven disorders, malaria was by far the leading killer over the ten-year period between 1897 and 1906. This is not surprising, given that the mosquito-borne disease was endemic throughout the island and occurred in all seasons. Morbidity and mortality due to malaria were thus a constant fact of life for many Taiwanese. Plague, however, occurred only episodically in certain subdistricts. The coefficient of variability for plague is therefore more than four times that of malaria.

Among the six other notifiable infectious diseases, plague was the leading cause of death between 1897 and 1906. On average, plague represented 3.65 percent of all causes of death between 1897 and 1906; the combined proportional mortality ratio of dysentery, smallpox, typhoid/typhus, diphtheria, and cholera represented less than 1 percent (see Table B.3). All five diseases resembled plague more than they did malaria in their pattern of variability. Of these epidemic diseases, cholera and smallpox were more episodic during this period than was plague, typhoid/typhus and dysentery occurred more consistently, and diphtheria had almost the same coefficient of variability.

Beginning in 1906, it is possible to compare statistics on plague mortality in Taiwan with all other causes of death (Table B.4). Although plague's proportional mortality ratio surpassed those of most other acute infectious diseases, the effects of plague were small relative to the more mundane, everyday causes of death. The majority of Taiwanese died from certain endemic transmissable diseases (malaria and tuberculosis), from respiratory ailments (pneumonia and bronchitis), from digestive disorders such as diarrhea (both infants and adults), during pregnancy or childbirth, and from "old age." Even accidental deaths (1.68 percent) accounted for a larger percentage of the total deaths over the ten-year period than did plague (0.80 percent). The coefficient of variability of plague was high relative to these more common, and constantly present, causes of death.

NOTES

Notes

INTRODUCTION

1. One exception to this statement is the work of Iijima Wataru (1991: 24–39). I am grateful to Professor Iijima for sending me copies of his study.

2. This discussion of plague epidemiology is based primarily on the work of Pollitzer and Meyer (1961: 433–501).

3. There is some controversy over whether the Southern China Commensal Rat Plague Focus constitutes a natural plague reservoir or is continually "replenished" from the Western Yunnan Transverse Valley reservoir. See Zhao Yongling (1982: 257) for a discussion of these two points of view.

4. The *Rattus flavipectus* species is found only in the tropical and subtropical regions of southern China and Southeast Asia. In China's tropical areas it represents between 60 and 95 percent of all commensal rodents, and in subtropical regions it constitutes some 20–80 percent of all rats. In temperate areas it makes up less than 6 percent of the total rodent population (Zhao Yongling 1982: 260). In contrast, the common brown rat (*Rattus norvegicus*) represents less than 7 percent of the rodent population in tropical China, 15–50 percent in subtropical regions, and 85–100 percent of all rats living in temperate areas. (Here "tropical" refers to an area where the average temperature ranges between 22 and 26°C and annual rainfall is between 1,500 and 2,500 mm. Subtropical regions are those with a January temperature of 0–15°C, a July temperature of 26–30°C, and annual rainfall 1,000–2,000 mm. Temperate climates are those where temperatures fall below 0°C in the winter.)

5. By the end of the nineteenth century, *shuyi* was being used by Chinese physicians to describe the disease identified by Western medicine as plague. See, for example, the 1891 treatise *Zhi shuyi fa* (Methods for curing plague), which I discuss at greater length in Chapter 4 (Zheng Xiaoyan 1936 [1901]:

preface). Some late-nineteenth-century gazetteer compilers used the term *shuyi* as well. See, for example, *Shanglinxian zhi* (1899 [1876], 1: 10a).

6. These issues present themselves not only to historians of disease but also to epidemiologists working in the present. The cause of the epidemic that broke out in India in the fall of 1994, widely reported to be pneumonic plague, remained controversial even two months after the epidemic ended. Some scientists disputed that the disease was plague because the plague bacterium had not yet been isolated in the laboratory. Others argued that it had to be plague because the classic symptoms and pathology of the pneunomic form of plague were evident in those afflicted (*New York Times*, Nov. 15, 1994: C3).

7. Wu Lien-teh, a self-described "plague fighter," was at the forefront of plague research and plague control efforts in China throughout the first half of the twentieth century. He was largely responsible for the establishment and ongoing operation of the Manchurian Plague Prevention Service, the earliest and most successful plague surveillance and control agency in China. For more on his work and life, see his autobiography (Wu 1959) and the brief biographical sketches presented by Fu Weikang (1984: 64–66) and Yang Shangchi (1988: 29–32).

1. ORIGINS OF PLAGUE

1. For examples of historical sources that discuss *zhangqi* (miasmas) and *yi* (epidemics) in Yunnan, see Li Yaonan (1954: 180) and Tian Jingguo (1987: 132).

2. Mention of *zhangqi* and *yi* can be found, for example, in *Dengchuanzhou zhi* (1853, 1: 5a), (*Xu*) *Yunnan tongzhigao* (1901, 2: 13b–24b), *Yongchangfu zhi* (1885, 1: 1a), and *Zhennanzhou zhi lue* (1892, 1: 44b). References to *zhangqi* are also common in many southwest China gazetteers, not just those for Yunnan. See, for example, in Guangxi province, *Nanningfu zhi* (1847, 3: 13b), and *Pinglefu zhi* (1805, 32: 3b–7b); and in Guizhou province, *Anshunfu zhi* (1851, 14: 7a), and *Xinyifu zhi* (1854, 5: 3a–3b). *Zhangqi* is commonly translated as "malaria," and no doubt many of the sources cited in these works describe malarial areas. Because *zhangqi* did not refer exclusively to malaria but included other febrile illnesses as well, I have chosen to translate it as "miasma."

3. For histories of malaria in Yunnan, see He Bin (1988); Li Yaonan (1954); and Ling, Liu, and Yao (1936).

4. Commensal rat plague foci are present in the following counties: (in Dali prefecture) Dali, Xiaguan, Xiangyun, Midu, and Weishan; (in Baoshan prefecture) Baoshan, Tengchong, Changning, Longling, Lianghe, Yingjiang, and Longchuan; and (in Dehong autonomous department) Ruili (Ji Shuli 1988: 47). The county names listed here are those currently in use in the People's Republic of China. Elsewhere in this study, I use place names current in the nineteenth century.

5. The nine other mammals responsible for plague transmission were found only in certain localities. They are: *Rattus sladeni* (Sladen's rat), *Mus musculus* (the common house mouse), *Rattus nitidus* (Himalayan rat), *Micromys minu-*

tus pygmaeus (Eurasian pygmy mouse), *Apodemus agrarius chevrieri* (Striped field mouse), *Eothenomys miletus* (Oriental vole), *Callosciurus erythraeus* (Belly-banded squirrel), *Crocidura attenuata* (a type of white-toothed shrew), and *Suncus murinus* (house shrew).

6. Although there are four types of fleas involved in plague transmission in Yunnan, the Asiatic rat flea (*Xenopsylla cheopis*) is the primary vector. The other three species are *Leptopsylla segnis*, *Monopsyllus anisus*, and *Paradoxopsyllus custodis*.

7. A similar danger exists in the American Southwest. The *New York Times* reports that the suburbanization of California, Arizona, and New Mexico has led to increased contact between house cats and plague-carrying rodents such as the deer mouse, rock squirrel, and the prairie dog. The newspaper notes that "Cats pick up the disease from infected fleas or rodents and pass it on when they bite, scratch, or lick humans. Even the breath of an infected cat, if it has mouth lesions, can transmit the plague bacteria" (*New York Times* May 8, 1994: A15). In 1993, out of the ten people who contracted bubonic plague, seven became infected at home, at least three by flea bites and two by contact with cats.

8. Twentieth-century studies of plague often mention Shi Daonan's poem, but these authors fail to cite its original source. Wu Lien-teh (1936: vii), for example, provides a translation of the poem but does not indicate its origin. The earliest version I have been able to find is the one included in Yuan Wenkui (1900 [1800], 21: 27b–29a). I would like to thank Yue Mingbao for providing a draft translation of the poem.

9. I am grateful to Susan Mann for her assistance in locating this reference.

10. *GZD I*, Gu Chun memorial "Zoubao Diannan liuxing bingzheng qingxing" (Report on the conditions of the epidemic in Yunnan province; Jiaqing 19/9/6 [1814] group 4, doc. 207–23). Gu Chun's (Gu Xihan) biography is included in *Qing shi liechuan* (1962, 73: 4a–5b). Yunnan was his first posting, at the age of twenty-two. His memorial reads as follows: "For more than ten years now, an epidemic has been spreading [*yi qi liuxing*] in Yunnan [Diannan]. People [with the disease] spit up blood, and on their bodies are lumps. The disease is customarily called *yangzi*. They die within two or three days. Last year and this year, this disease has been prevalent in the area of Lin'an. No fewer than one hundred thousand people have died. Those who suffer from this disease are all a pitiful sight. There is nothing worse than this. No one I visited recognized its origins. Those skilled with drugs can only prescribe cold or hot medicine. None have any effect. I have already collected and distributed rare medicine. Some was effective, some was not. Now the epidemic is lessening in intensity but it has not yet stopped throughout the entire province." (The figure one hundred thousand cannot be taken literally but should be read as "a very great number.")

11. *Yangzibing* is the name often used in gazetteer accounts as well. See, for example, (*Xu*) *Mengzixian zhi* (1961 [1911], 12: 43b) and (*Xuxiu*) *Jianshuixian zhigao* (1920, 10: 22a).

12. By "Yungui region" I mean the geographical territory that encompasses

the major river systems of Yunnan and Guizhou provinces and includes a small part of southern Sichuan as demarcated by G. William Skinner (1977b: 241); see also my Maps 1 and 2. Although Susan Naquin and Evelyn Rawski (1987: 199) call this region Southwest China, I prefer to use Skinner's original terminology. James Lee (1993: 1) also uses the term "Southwest China," but his boundaries for this region differ slightly from those drawn by Skinner. I am grateful to Professor Lee for sharing with me a manuscript copy of his "State and Economy in Southwest China, 1250–1850."

13. For descriptions of areas that boomed following the opening of mines, see *Mengzixian zhi* (1797 [1791], 3: 45a) and *Pu'erfu zhigao* (1900, 11: 2b and 20: 31a).

14. Road construction on most of the major routes in the southwest began in the thirteenth century under the Mongols (J. Lee 1993: 94). During the Ming period, some roads were paved with stones. Ferries and bridges (stone, suspension, and pontoon) were also in use at that time (Lombard-Salmon 1972: 96–98). After the Muslim Rebellion (1856–73), the roads of the province were in very bad shape. Nonetheless, late-nineteenth-century European travelers described a paved road system that must have been quite extensive at one time. See Carné (1982 [1872]: 223–25, 231, 240, 266, 324) and Gill (1883: 242).

15. See James Lee's manuscript (1993: 92–94; 331–37) for a concise summary of the six major routes leading to southwestern China in use between 1250 and 1850. I include two routes not discussed by Lee, the one from Dali to Tibet and the one from Laos to Kunming. See Prasertkul (1989: 13–14) for an excellent description of trade routes in use in the late nineteenth century.

16. Each of these trade routes was "explored" in the late nineteenth century by Europeans searching for a commercial route into China from Burma or Indochina. See Cooper (1871b: 271–452) and Gill (1883: 224–318) for descriptions of the Adunzi-Lijiang-Dali and Dali-Tengyue-Burma routes. The French expedition to explore the Mekong under Doudart de Lagrée and Francis Garnier followed the route from Laos to Simao and Kunming (Carné 1982 [1872]: 212–365). Intent on visiting Dali, they took a circuitous detour along the Jinsha River to western Yunnan. Finally, upon returning to eastern Yunnan, they followed the imperial route used to transport Yunnan's minerals to the interior into Sichuan and down the Yangzi River. Archibald Colquhoun (1883) went up West River tributaries as far as Bose and then traveled to Simao through southeastern Yunnan. He then went to Dali from Simao by way of Jingdong. Each of these accounts provides fascinating details on the topography, commerce, and settlements along each road.

17. Salt was the main commodity transported within the province; the road between the largest saltwells in the province (Baiyanjing) and Kunming was heavily traveled. Cotton was imported from Burma; by 1838, 30 million pounds of Burmese cotton were being transported annually into Yunnan (T'ien 1982: 24). Pu'er tea from Xishuangbanna was highly desired in both Tibet and the interior of China. Dali was famous for its marble, and Yunnan's mines provided the rest of the empire not only with copper but also with zinc, lead, and

tin. Nanning county in Qujing prefecture was the center of lead production; the most important lead mines in the province were located in Zhanyi department (Hosie 1890: 50). (Nanning later became renowned as an area where high-grade opium was grown [Inspectorate General, *Decennial Reports* 1882–91: 669].) Dongchuan prefecture was the center of the copper mining industry, and the most productive tin mines were situated in the Gejiu district of Lin'an prefecture.

18. A natural plague focus is also known to exist on the Qinghai-Tibetan Plateau, and plague may very well have originally been imported into the Lijiang area from Tibet (Ji Shuli 1988: 65).

19. From eastern Yunnan, this epidemic may have spread as far as Xinyi county (1808), Anshun prefecture (1815) and Anping county (1824) in Guizhou province (Guizhousheng tushuguan 1982: 378–79). It may also have spread to Shanglin and Binzhou in Guangxi. Both of these county-level units are located along the Yunnan-Canton West River trade route and both recorded large epidemics for the year 1810 (*Binzhou zhi* 1826, 23: 6a; *Shanglinxian zhi* 1899 [1876], 1: 8a). Shanglin did have an outbreak of plague (*shuyi*) in 1867 (*Shanglinxian zhi* 1899 [1876], 1: 10a), but the descriptions of the 1810 epidemics in both Shanglin and Binzhou are too vague to say with any certainty whether or not they were linked to the Yunnan plague. (See Chapter 2 for discussion of the 1867 Shanglin epidemic.)

20. The compilation on the history of plague in China prepared by the Chinese Academy of Medical Sciences (*SYLXS*) lists many more plague epidemics for the nineteenth century than I do here. The lists in that work were prepared following what is termed "investigations" conducted in the early 1950's. The compilers of the Yunnan section of this collection were not clear about what method (oral histories, local archival research, or epidemiological studies) they used. In the absence of written records to verify these investigations, I have chosen not to include them here. Anyone interested in seeing the results of these reports may refer to my dissertation (Benedict 1992: 74, 87–90, 96–97, 100, 104–6).

21. The chronic problem of underregistration in the official population registers was no doubt exacerbated by the civil war, and these figures are almost certainly inaccurate.

22. Rocher's notes on the Yunnan plague were widely cited by his nineteenth-century contemporaries (e.g., Inspectorate General, *Customs Medical Reports* 1877–78, No. 15: 25–27) and in subsequent historical and epidemiological studies (Pollitzer 1954; Simpson 1905: 48–66; Wong and Wu 1935: 508). It was his observations that allowed nineteenth-century epidemiologists to identify Yunnan as the probable starting point of the third pandemic of plague.

23. See Rocher's map for locations where plague outbreaks were most intense (1879, 2: map folder).

24. For descriptions of population decline in the Dali region due to the rebellion, see *Dalixian zhigao* (1917, 3: 7a) and *Menghua xianxiang tuzhi* (n.d., Guangxu edition, *hukou* [population] section).

25. For a similar description of the plague, see (*Xuxiu*) *Jianshuixian zhigao* (1920, 10: 22a).

2. INTERREGIONAL SPREAD

1. The Lingnan macroregion, defined largely by the drainage basin of the West River system, encompasses most of the territory of Guangxi and Guangdong (Skinner 1977b: 212); see my Maps 1 and 2.

2. Tonkin was the northern part of French Indochina (Vietnam), with Hanoi (Chin. *Dongjing*; Viet. *Tongking*) as its capital. By using "Tonkin" rather than "Vietnam," I am both giving the nineteenth-century designation and stressing the border region between China and Vietnam, rather than Annam, which is farther south.

3. The Leizhou Peninsula now falls within the provincial boundaries of Guangxi, but in the nineteenth century it was administratively part of Guangdong (Tan Qixiang 1980, 8: 44–45).

4. The West (Xi) River system originates in Yunnan, passes through Guangxi and parts of Guangdong, and empties into the Pearl River Delta. The two main tributaries in the upper course of the system are the You River (which flows east from Guangnan in Yunnan) and the Zuo River (which originates in Tonkin). These meet at Nanning to form the Yu River. At Guiping county the Yu River joins the Hongshui River, and from Guiping to Wuzhou the river is called the Xun. The section known as the West River begins in Wuzhou. In the eighteenth century, the West River route was used primarily to transport copper from eastern Yunnan to Canton (Laai 1950: 88–89). Salt from western Guangdong was also transported into Yunnan along this route.

5. In the 1880's Yunnan opium sold in Bose at $345 per picul (one picul is the weight one man can carry, and ranges between 102 and 133 lb.) had increased to $395 per picul by the time it reached Longzhou (Inspectorate General, *Decennial Reports* 1882–91: 655). This contrasted with $600 per picul of Patna opium from India sold in Longzhou. In Beihai, Patna opium cost Hong Kong taels (HK.Tls) 395; Yunnan opium cost HK.Tls 165 (ibid.: 642).

6. Lin Manhong's (1985) doctoral dissertation is the most comprehensive study of domestically grown opium during the Qing period. For a discussion of opium cultivation and the Yunnan-Lingnan opium trade in the late nineteenth century, see Metzgar (1973: 20–22). The Yunnan-Lingnan opium trade down the West River system in the Republican era is discussed by Lary (1974: 44, 92, 190).

7. Shi Fan, an eighteenth-century Yunnanese official, discusses both the Kunming–Guangnan and the Kunming–Luoping roads in his description of merchant routes in Yunnan (1891a, 11: 6049–50). For a description of the river passage from Canton to Bose, see Colquhoun (1883, vol. 1) and Tōa Dōbunkai (1919, 2: 434–44).

8. In 1890, on the order of 1,000,000 kg (an estimated 18,000 piculs) of

opium were transported from Yunnan down the You River to Nanning along this route (Inspectorate General, *Decennial Reports* 1882–91: 655).

9. The Red River route was by far the shortest and most rapid route between Yunnan and Canton after steamship travel became possible in the second half of the nineteenth century. Overland from Kunming to the border town of Manhao took eleven days, and the trip down the Red River took sixteen days (Royal Asiatic Society 1893–94: 75). By ocean steamer, the trip from Haiphong to Hong Kong took only two days (ibid.: 61). The route had been used before the Muslim Rebellion to transport opium and tin, but during the 1860's banditry along the upper reaches of the Red River largely disrupted legalized trade. Regular commerce along the river did not really pick up again until the last two decades of the nineteenth century.

10. In addition to Pingxiang, there were two other border crossings suitable for large groups and numerous points where small caravans could pass. See Laffey (1976: 70–71, fn. 18) for sources that describe various routes along the Sino-Vietnamese frontier in use during the nineteenth century.

11. Laai (1950: 62–73) discusses in detail the history of Cantonese river pirates in Guangxi and the historical reasons for their migration into Guangxi. Laai, Michael, and Sherman (1962) describe the many river pirate bands that existed in the province between 1840 and 1870. See articles by Laffey (1972; 1975; and 1976) on the bandits that operated along the Sino-Vietnamese border during the same period. On the Qinzhou sea pirates who preyed on commercial and fishing junks in the Gulf of Tonkin early in the century, see Murray (1987: 6–20). Wakeman (1966: 117–48; 1972) discusses mid-nineteenth-century triad activity in Guangdong and Guangxi.

12. Beihai's position on the main trade corridors of western peripheral Lingnan made it the premier choice of foreign powers when they sought a site for a treaty port in western Guangdong. After Beihai was opened to foreign trade in 1876, the town grew rapidly, and by 1891 it had an estimated population of 25,000 (Inspectorate General, *Decennial Reports* 1882–91: 645).

13. I have been unable to verify the date or purpose of Beihai's establishment with other sources. The settlement does not appear on maps included in either the 1833 Lianzhou prefectural gazetteer or in the 1864 edition of the Guangdong provincial gazetteer (*Guangdong tongzhi* 1864; *Lianzhoufu zhi* 1833). It is included on the map of Hepu county in the *Guangdong yudi quanshuo* (Complete explication of the atlas of Guangdong; see Liao Tingxiang 1967 [1889], 7: 3b) and in the late Qing edition of *Guangdong yudi quantu* (Comprehensive atlas of Guangdong; Zhang Renqun 1967 [1897]: n.p.). The 1813 edition of the *Da Qing huidian* (Statutes of the Qing dynasty) lists Lianzhou as a customs collections station but fails to mention Beihai; the 1899 edition adds Beihai as a prefectural-level collectorate (cited in Cushman 1975: 34). This may, however, simply reflect the increased prominence of Beihai due to its designation as a treaty port after 1876.

14. Xie Xingyao (1950: 223–30) includes a chronological list of anti-Qing

military activity organized by place. According to this listing, territory along the Yunnan-Beihai trade routes in Guangxi and western Guangdong was not militarized until the late 1850's.

15. For descriptions of continued opium cultivation in Yunnan in the 1860's, see Cooper (1871b: 323, 335) and Carné (1982 [1872]: 309).

16. See Colquhoun (1883, vol. 1) for a description of the ubiquity of *lijin* collection depots along the West River in 1882.

17. After plague first appeared on the Leizhou Peninsula in the early 1870's, the disease continued to occur almost annually until 1952 in Suixi, Zhanjiang, and Leizhou (*SYLXS* 1982: 1490, 1570, and 1576).

3. PLAGUE IN THE SOUTHEAST

1. The Southeast Coast contains the basins of four river systems: the Ou, the Min, the Jiulong, and the Han Rivers. All of Fujian province falls within its borders, as do sections of northeastern Guangdong and southeastern Zhejiang (Skinner 1985: 277); see also my Maps 1 and 2.

2. The classic study of innovation diffusion was done by Torsten Hägerstrand (1967 [1953]). Following his pioneering efforts, a large body of geographical scholarship has developed on spatial diffusion. For an introduction to Hägerstrand's work and subsequent diffusion studies, see Bradford and Kent (1989 [1977]: 128–42).

3. Economic geographers use the term "contagious" to describe this type of diffusion, but since some noncontagious diseases also spread in this way, medical geographers prefer the term "contact" or "expansion" to avoid confusion.

4. In an analysis of cholera diffusion in Africa in the early 1970's, Stock (1976) illustrated how cholera spread both through contact diffusion and in an urban-hierarchical fashion in the same area. One or the other pattern was followed in the initial stages of an epidemic; this phase was followed by a secondary stage where the other pattern obtained. Moreover, he identified three types of contact diffusion: coastal (where the coast served as the primary diffusion channel and location on the coast was the most important variable); riverine (where river valleys served as the primary diffusion channel and location on the river was the most important variable); and radial (where the lack of prominent urban centers and the absence of natural barriers or channels allowed the infection to spread out evenly from a central source).

5. Relocation diffusion alone tends to occur in industrialized societies where there is a well-developed system of mechanized transport. Pyle (1969) studied the diffusion of three major cholera epidemics in the United States in the nineteenth century. The first (introduced in 1832) spread along waterways in the eastern part of the country to both urban and rural areas. The second (1849) occurred when railroads were becoming increasingly important but had not yet replaced canals and rivers as the major transport corridors. As a result, cholera reached many agricultural areas. The third epidemic (1866) started after the railway system was well established, and diffusion during

this wave was clearly structured on the country's urban hierarchy. Cholera spread rapidly from one city to another along the transportation system and bypassed large segments of the rural hinterland altogether.

6. As discussed in the Introduction, the yellow-chested rat is the predominant commensal rodent species in China's tropical and subtropical climates; the common brown rat is more numerous in temperate areas. In studies done in the 1950's, 70 percent of the rats trapped in Quanzhou were yellow-chested rats. In 1957 in Shantou, *Rattus flavipectus* represented 58 percent of all rats caught, while *Rattus norvegicus* represented only 41 percent and the common house mouse (*Mus musculus*) less than 1 percent. Farther north, in Wenzhou, the brown rat was more common than the yellow-chested rat (*SYLXS* 1982: 1703). In China plague is more commonly seen in areas where the yellow-chested rat predominates.

7. Wenzhou is an exception. Plague did not appear there until 1943, after it had already spread from Fujian to other towns in the interior of Zhejiang. That Wenzhou exhibits a different pattern of diffusion underscores the fact that, although plague tends to follow human movement, it remains conditioned by natural and environmental factors. Conditions in three areas of the macro-region (Xiamen, Fuzhou, and Shantou) are favorable for the *Rattus flavipectus* plague host. The area around Wenzhou is less hospitable to the rat, and thus plague appeared there later and with much less frequency than it did in the subregions further south. Its arrival in the 1940's is most probably linked to wartime migrations.

8. In three of these subregions (Xiamen, Yanping, and Shantou), the disease arrived first in the regional city (Xiamen in 1884, Shantou in 1894, and Yanping in 1900); in the case of Fuzhou, plague appeared in smaller-order centers (Putian and Xianyou) before it arrived in the regional city.

9. This analysis is very crude in the sense that it assumes a process of diffusion between individual settlements but takes the county as the basic unit of analysis because that is how the data are presented in the source consulted (*SYLXS* 1982: 931–1454). Plague often spread across county borders in ways that are lost when diffusion processes are aggregated to the county level. Moreover, because I have information only on the year and not the month in which the disease first appeared in a particular county or settlement, it is impossible to trace the diffusion of the disease through time and space in a highly sophisticated way. The patterns of diffusion described here are those that make most sense to me based on what I know of the human geography of the region, and should be read as probabilistic rather than certain.

10. The Xiamen regional-city trading system included the following counties: Haicheng, Tongan, Longxi, Nanjing, Zhangping, Huian, Nan'an, Jinjiang, Anxi, Zhangpu, Yongchun, Changtai, Hua'an, and Longyan. In this system and those considered later, I only discuss counties with reported plague epidemics. I have not adhered perfectly to the boundaries used by Skinner because in certain instances county boundaries are dissected by trading system boundaries. Counties whose borders cross over regional-city trading sys-

tem boundaries are included in the system that incorporates the most territory.

11. The 1887 peak is due largely to a reported 7,800 deaths in Zhangzhou city (*SYLXS* 1982: 1010). This figure seems highly suspicious because it was never replicated following the 1887 outbreak. Zhangzhou had frequent plague outbreaks from 1889 to 1947, but with the exception of 1932, when 5,800 people reportedly died from the disease, the estimated number of fatalities from plague in the city was consistently listed as below 100.

12. This graph includes both suburban areas outside of Zhangzhou, Xiamen, and Quanzhou and rural villages.

13. The Fuzhou regional-city trading system included the following counties: Putian, Xianyou, Fuqing, Pingtan, Houguan, Yongfu, Lianjiang, Gutian, Ningde, Zhoudun, Luoyuan, Changle, Xiapu, Datian, and Minqing.

14. Shantou's regional-city system incorporated the following counties: Meizhou, Xingning, Raoping, Dapu, Huilai, Puning, Haifeng, Chaoyang, Lufeng, Pinghe, Chenghai, Jieyang, Fengshun, Wuhua, Zhenping, Pingyuan, Dongshan, Zhaoan, Yongding, and Yunxiao. The data in *SYLXS* for the Shantou regional-city trading system are much less comprehensive than are materials for the three other regional-city trading systems I discuss in this chapter. I am therefore unable to graph the numbers of deaths or the number of villages affected for the Shantou subregion.

15. Counties in the Yanping regional-city trading system included Shaxian, Nanping, Jian'an, Jianyang, Chongan, Pucheng, Shunchang, Zhenghe, Pingnan (only a portion), Songxi, Yongan, Shaowu, Guangze, Taining, Jiangle, and Youxi.

4. NINETEENTH-CENTURY RESPONSES

1. Along with other modern scholars, I use the term "classical Chinese medicine" to refer only to the literate tradition of the scholarly elite and not to more widespread folk practices of healing. For more on this distinction, see Sivin (1987: 22).

2. Judith Farquhar (1994: 61–135) discusses the five diagnostic techniques most commonly used in Chinese medical clinics today. These are the eight rubrics (*ba gang*) analysis, illness factor (*bingyin*) analysis, visceral systems (*zangfu*), and the two discussed here, four sectors (*wei qi ying xue*) analysis, and six warps (*liu jing*) analysis.

3. The best explication in English of these classical Chinese medical concepts is that of Sivin (1987: 43–94). Sivin notes that the five phases and the six warps are best understood as subcategories of the *yinyang* polarity and that all three concepts serve as labels of *qi*, "the basic stuff." Each of the five phases and six warps corresponds to a particular season of the year, underscoring the importance of seasonality in Chinese medical thinking.

4. The *Huangdi neijing*, or *Neijing*, remains the basic canon of classical Chinese medicine because it introduces the concepts that form the theoretical underpinnings of the Chinese medical system. Structured as a dialogue be-

tween the legendary Yellow Emperor and his ministers, it is actually a collection of medical treatises written by different authors over the course of a hundred years or more, and was probably brought together in the first century B.C.E. For a summary of *Neijing* scholarship, see Sivin (1993).

5. The seven emotional states (joy, anger, melancholy, anxiety, sorrow, fear, and fright) are considered to be internal factors that can cause illness when felt in excess.

6. In linking atmospheric conditions and the weather to ill health, the Cold Damage lineage continues a tradition established much earlier. "Wind" and "snow" appear in Shang oracle bones as important illness factors, although it is not entirely clear whether the inscriptions are referring to natural or supernatural phenomena (Unschuld 1985: 25). A famous passage in the *Zuo zhuan* (Commentary of Zuo, fifth-fourth century B.C.E.) identifies six types of *qi* (*yin*, *yang*, wind, rain, darkness, and light) that, in excess, cause six categories of illness (Sivin 1987: 55). These six *qi* are conceptually distinct from the *liu qi* (six climatic configurations) that later became important in etiological thinking. As Shigehisa Kuriyama notes (1993: 55; 1994: 23–41), the conception of illness as a seasonal phenomenon emerged most clearly in the Han period.

7. The following discussion of the Warm Factor tradition draws on a number of studies, including Deng Tietao (1955); Farquhar (1994); Gao Hesheng (1979); Gou Qianheng (1985); Hanson (1991); Shi Changyong (1957); and Shi Yiren (1955). Marta Hanson's forthcoming dissertation (University of Pennsylvania) promises to present a sophisticated and comprehensive history of the Warm Factor school.

8. See the annotated version of the *Wenyi lun* published by Zhejiangsheng zhongyi yanjiusuo (1976).

9. For discussion of the theories of Ye Tianshi and Wu Jutong, see Gao Hesheng (1979) and Zhao Yi (1979).

10. Warm Factor explanations of plague etiology and the therapeutic practices designed to combat it appear to have won widespread popular acceptance at the turn of the century. Unlike Huang Zhongxian's treatise, which quickly faded into obscurity, Luo Rulan's *Shuyi huibian* (Compilation on plague) went through five printings between 1891 and 1897. Sixteen hundred copies of the fifth edition were sponsored by two benevolent associations (*shantang*) and distributed to native-place organizations around Guangdong. *Shuyi yuebian* also appears to have circulated widely throughout the southeast. Charitable societies in Fujian paid to have the work reproduced and distributed to local communities (Luoyuanxian weiyuan hui 1985: 112). Zheng Xiaoyan's recommended prescriptions were also recorded in numerous gazetteers (*Guixian zhi* 1935, 18: 586; *Yangjiangxian zhi* 1925, 37: 44), and the entire treatise was reprinted in a 1936 compilation of famous Chinese medical works (Zheng Xiaoyan 1936 [1901], 7: 1–66). Brief biographies of Wu Zongxuan, Luo Rulan, and Zheng Xiaoyan appear in *Zhongyi renwu cidian* (Dictionary of notable figures in Chinese medicine; Zhongyi yanjiuyuan 1988: 252, 385, and 415). On Wu Zongxuan, see also the entry in *Wuchuanxian zhi* (1892 [1888], 6: 54a); Luo Rulan's biography is included in *Shichengxian zhi* (1892, 6: 28b–29a).

11. For a more detailed discussion of varied religious beliefs and practices during epidemics, see Paul Katz's 1990 dissertation. Katz describes in impressive detail the history of beliefs surrounding the Five Commissioners of Epidemics; a number of *wenshen* (plague god) cults, including that of Wen Yuanshuai; and the *wenshen jiao*, rituals and processionals used both to prevent and to expel epidemics.

12. For another description of vengeful plague ghosts that caused epidemic disease, see the poems "Yigui" (Plague ghosts) by Yuan Tang and "Zhu Yigui" (Expelling the plague ghosts) by Tang Sunhua. Both are included in Zhang Yingchang (1960 [1875], 2: 896, 879).

13. There is a growing body of literature on the beliefs and practices surrounding the worship of plague gods on Taiwan. In addition to the work of Liu Zhiwan (1962; 1966; 1983) and Paul Katz (1987; 1990; 1991), see Kristofer M. Schipper (1985) and Sung Kwang-yu (1990: chap. 5).

14. Historical descriptions of *wenshen* rituals used to appease or exorcise plague deities can be found in the following gazetteers: in Guangxi province, *Shanglinxian zhi* (1899 [1876], 2: 12b); in Yunnan province, *Dataoxian zhi* (1845, 2: 56b), *Dengchuanzhou zhi* (1853, 4: 6a), *Jingdongfu zhi* (1732, 1: n.p.), *Maguanxian zhi* (1932, 2: n.p.), *Pu'erfu zhi* (1850 [1840], 9: 3a), and *Yaozhou zhi* (1885, 1: 32b); and in Guizhou province, *Bijiexian zhi* (1879, 7: 9a), and *Dadingfu zhi* (1849, 14: 20b).

15. Guan Yu (162–220 C.E.) received the imperial title *di* in 1615. Most popularly known as the God of War, Guandi was adopted as a patron god and protector by many different social groups. Prasenjit Duara (1988b) analyzes the many official and nonofficial images of Guandi.

16. Detailed descriptions of *wenshen jiao* and the exorcistic processionals associated with them are provided by Paul Katz (1990: 178–214) and Francis Hsu (1952). *Jiao* have many purposes other than epidemic prevention or expulsion, of course. This discussion is limited to those performed expressly to rid a community of epidemic ghosts or gods.

17. Liu Zhiwan quotes a passage from Xie Zhaozhi's *Wuzazu* (Five Miscellanies) that describes the plague boats in Fujian during the Ming period: "In Fujian . . . the spirit mediums use paper to make a boat which is put on the water. The people worship this boat and every night they take it out. The residents all close their windows against it. In the night, they carry the boat into the countryside; those who meet it along the way do not look at it" (Liu Zhiwan 1983: 287). The ritual as it is practiced today in Xigang (in Tainan county, Taiwan) is described by Liu Zhiwan (ibid.: 285–400) and Paul Katz (1987: 198–99). See Katz (1990: 196–203) for a description of boat-burning rituals in Zhejiang.

18. In his study of the Dragon Boat Festival in Hunan and Hubei, Göran Aijmer (1964: 57–58, 92–93) uncovered many references from the *Gujin tushu ji cheng* (Complete collection of writings and illustrations, past and present) which indicate that the high points of the Duanwu (Dragon Boat Festival) were the *songwen* ("escorting epidemics") or *zhu yi* ("driving out epidemics") rituals, both of which involved the burning of grass or paper plague boats.

James Hayes (1983: 153–64) describes similar ceremonies in central Guang-dong in which *caolongchuan* (which he translates as "Dragon Boats on Land") were ritually burnt or allowed to float away in order to dispel disease and pla-cate the plague gods.

19. Other gazetteers also describe *Qing jiao* designed specifically to prevent epidemics: in Yunnan province, *Jingdong zhiliting zhi* (1788, 3: 1b); in Guizhou province, *Sinanfu xu zhi* (1841, 2: 30a), *Suiyangxian zhi* (1928, 1: 16a), *Xingrenxian bu zhi* (1943, 14: 16a–16b), and (*Zengxiu*) *Renhuaiting zhi* (1902, 6: 35b); and in Guangxi province, *Longzhou jilue* (1803, *fengsu* [customs] section). Francis Hsu (1952: 20–24) describes this ritual following an outbreak of epidemic cholera in Yunnan in 1942. An elderly man told Hsu (ibid.: 67) that the same ritual had been performed on a large scale twenty-three years earlier, and it seems likely that it was performed in the nineteenth century as well. The burning of *wenshen* boats is mentioned in a Guizhou prefectural gazetteer, so the ritual was performed historically at least in some parts of the southwest (*Dadingfu zhi* 1849, 14: 20b).

20. Bao Gong was also appealed to by the Chinese community in Macao during the 1895 plague outbreak there (Hayes 1977: 66).

21. An American missionary living in Shantou (Swatow) reported in 1901 that many communities only began to experience plague after *wenshen* fes-tivals attracted crowds from the surrounding towns and villages that were already infected. See NA, USDS, RG 59, M101, McWade to Hill, reel 15, no. 113, June 25, 1901.

22. This type of guard system was common in the northeast as well. During the 1910–11 plague epidemic in Manchuria, villages would not allow strangers to enter and built walls to isolate infected neighborhoods (*NCH* Mar. 3, 1911: 488, and Apr. 1, 1911: 26). It is not clear when this practice of building walls during epidemics began.

23. Children wore girdles filled with realgar around their waist or cords treated with the substance around their ankles and wrists. Some parents put dots of realgar on their children's foreheads or even bathed their children in it. Satchels filled with realgar were hung around the neck and placed under the nostrils when noxious smells were encountered. Gazetteers describing the use of charms treated with realgar on Duanwu include: in Guangxi province, *Binzhou zhi* (1886, 19: 3a) and *Shanglinxian zhi* (1899 [1876], 2: 12a); in Guizhou province, *Xingrenxian zhi* (1934, 9: 12b); and in Yunnan province, *Dengchuan-zhou zhi* (1853: 4b–5a), *Jingdong zhiliting zhi* (1788, 3: n.p.), and *Tengyuezhou zhi* (1790, 3: 25b).

24. A 1641 treatise written by Hu Zhengxin advocates boiling the clothes of victims of epidemic disease (Lee 1958: 190). See also Xia Yihuang (1935) on the custom of burning the clothing of the deceased as a preventive health measure.

25. NA, USDS, RG 59, M101, McWade to Hill, reel 15, no. 113, June 25, 1901.

26. For the historian of disease, the paucity of official reports is frustrating enough, but it posed very real problems for Qing officials seeking precedents on which to base their relief efforts during epidemics. The statecraft writer

Yuan Yixiang, writing in 1660, complained that "the honored precedents discuss disasters, but . . . they are limited to earthquakes, droughts, floods and
that kind of thing . . . they do not extend to epidemics. [When] referring to the
Huidian [Statutes] one always comes across mention of disasters, . . . but . . .
no matter if they are large or small, all are floods, droughts, and famines" (He
Changling 1886, 45: 2a–2b).

27. For descriptions of *tenghuang* (yellow notices) posted after epidemics,
see *GZD II*, Gui Fang and Peng Ling memorial, Jiaqing 19/3/22 (1814), group
359-4-75, box 78; and ibid., Qing Bao memorial, Jiaqing 19/3/30 (1814), group
359-4-75, box 78.

28. Tax-payment deferral following an epidemic is described in *GZD II*,
anonymous, "Yunnan yili liuxing qingxing" (The condition of the epidemic
spreading in Yunnan), Guangxu 15 (1889), group 359-4-75, box 89.

29. Descriptions of such donations can be found in *GZD I*, anonymous,
"Zouwei Guzhouzhen liuxing chuanran bingzheng" (A report on the disease
spreading through Guzhouzhen), Qianlong 12/10 (1747), group 4, doc. 207.8;
ibid., Zhang Shicheng enclosure, Daoguang 1/9/3 (1821), group 4, doc. 207.26;
and ibid., Zhang Shicheng memorial, Daoguang 1/9/15 (1821), group 4, doc.
207.27.

30. This Kunming dispensary was established at the beginning of the Jiaqing
reign (1796–1820) after two provincial-level degree-holders (*juren*) collected
subscriptions from local gentry in the area (*Kunmingxian zhi* 1939, 2: 13a–14b).
(See also the charitable pharmacy described in [*Xuxiu*] *Yongbei zhiliting zhi*
1904, 2: 13b.) State administrators appear to have taken a relatively active role
in the establishment and ongoing management of charitable agencies in Yunnan. The Yungui governor-general and the Yunnan governor established the
Kunming county poorhouse (*puji tang*) in 1726, two years after the Yongzheng
emperor ordered the empirewide establishment of *puji tang* (Leung 1987: 148).
After the poorhouse was destroyed in the mid-nineteenth century, during
the Muslim Rebellion, the governor-general took the initiative to have it re-
built (*Kunmingxian zhi* 1939, 2: 1a–1b). For more on charitable dispensaries, see
Leung (1987) and Lum (1985).

31. A military doctor in Yunnan during the Qianlong reign, for example,
personally gave out congé and free medicine during epidemic outbreaks there
(*Yongchangfu zhi* 1826, 50: 1b). On the official solicitation of private donations,
see *GZD II*, Gui Fang and Peng Ling memorial, Jiaqing 19/3/22 (1814), group
359-4-75, box 78.

32. During the Ming-Qing period, the *Taiyiyuan* (Imperial Medical Bureau)
was primarily responsible for treating the emperor and his dependents, but
Taiyiyuan physicians also treated high-ranking officials, foreigners staying in
the capital, and prison wardens (Gong Chun 1959). *Taiyiyuan* doctors were
occasionally sent to the provinces to treat officials and soldiers stationed in the
field (Yunnansheng lishi yanjiusuo 1984, 4: 729). An important function of the
Imperial Medical Bureau was the collection, preparation, and distribution of
medicinal herbs. Local officials sent efficacious remedies to the Board of Rites

(*Libu*), which passed them on to the *Taiyiyuan* for storage. The drugs were recorded in two record books, one kept by the Medical Bureau, the other by the Board of Rites (Gong Chun 1960: 223).

33. A request that "peace and harmony" (*ping'an dan*) pills be sent from Beijing to Sichuan is found in *GZD I*, Liu Binggua memorial, Qianlong 40/1/19 (1775), group 4, doc. 207.13. A similar request is that of ibid., anonymous, "Zouqing enyang biwen difang yijiu difang shiyi pian" (Enclosure requesting the compassionate [distribution] of remedies to rescue localities from epidemic disease), no date, group 4, doc. 207.46.

34. *Awei*, the subject of these memorials, was probably asafetida (*Ferula assafoetida*), the resin of a tree found in Persia and northern India. For a description of *awei* and its application in Chinese medicine, see P. Smith (1969: 173–74) and Hirth and Rockhill (1911, 2: 224). James Duke (1985: 194) describes the chemical properties of asafetida and its current uses.

35. Street cleaning in the wake of epidemics appears to have been a common practice. See, for example, Lao Tong's (1935–40 [1794], vol. 969, 4: 47) advice on this subject in *Jiuhuang beilan* (Materials for famine administration).

36. Burial of victims of any calamity, not just epidemics, was often a governmental responsibility. Officially sponsored charitable graveyards were commonplace and were used for the poor and indigent as well as for victims of disaster. See Lum (1985: 142–43).

37. In Baiyanjing, for example, it was believed that the improper burial of plague victims in 1854 generated further outbreaks because the corpses gave off heteropathic *qi* (*xie qi*; see *Yanfengxian zhi* 1924, 2.2: 1153).

38. For brief descriptions of European and Middle Eastern responses to plague, see the essays by Ann Carmichael and Katharine Park in the *Cambridge World History of Human Disease* (Carmichael 1993: 628–31; Park 1993: 612–16). Indian reactions to plague in the nineteenth and early twentieth centuries might be added here as yet another example of the similarity of responses to the disease within different cultures (Arnold 1993: 200–39). The following sample of headlines indicates that many of the same responses were evident during the 1994 outbreak of pneumonic plague in India: "Thousands Flee Indian City in Deadly Plague Outbreak" (*New York Times* Sept. 24, 1994: A1); "Rumors Fuel Plague Panic in India" (*Washington Post* Sept. 26, 1994: A16); and "Plague Turns India into Region's Pariah" (*Washington Post* Oct. 2, 1994: A29).

5. PLAGUE IN CANTON AND HONG KONG

1. I have been unable to find any specific official report of the 1894 plague outbreak in Canton. Li Hanzhang was the governor-general of Guangdong and Guangxi at the time but makes no mention of the epidemic in his collected papers (Li Hanzhang 1967 [1900]). The governor of Guangdong was the notorious Manchu conservative, Gangyi. Many of Gangyi's memorials regarding the state of affairs in Guangdong in 1894 are reprinted in *Gongzhongdang Guangxuchao zouzhe* (1973–75, vol. 8), but none record the plague epidemic. Brief

descriptions of the epidemic in Canton are included in the Nanhai and Panyu county gazetteers (*Nanhaixian zhi* 1910, 2: 69a; *Panyuxian xu zhi* 1931, 44: 8).

2. Similar regulations regarding the transport of nightsoil were in effect in other Chinese cities, such as Shanghai, Fuzhou, and Hankou (Rowe 1989: 170).

3. The "Jêntsi" (Renji *shantang*) is described in *Panyuxian xu zhi* (1931, 5: 27); the "Kuangtsi" (Guangji *shantang*) is mentioned in *Nanhaixian zhi* (1910, 6: 11b). The "Tungshan" was probably the Tong *shantang* (ibid.: 13a). It is not clear what "Szemiao" refers to.

4. Many similar complaints can be found in the writings of foreign missionaries and consular officials. See, for example, NA, PHS, RG 90, Central File, C. Johnson to A. Johnson, no. 5608, box 639, Feb. 12, 1900; and NA, USDS, RG 59, M101, McWade to Hill, reel 15, no. 118, July 3, 1901.

5. The Donghua Hospital replaced an ancestral hall that had served as a hospice and as a coffin repository for Cantonese sojourners in the colony since 1851. Although the Hong Kong government provided a site for the hospital and some financial support, most of the money for the hospital came from the voluntary contributions of wealthy Chinese. Studies of the Donghua Hospital Directorate and its leadership role in nineteenth-century Hong Kong include Lethbridge (1978), Sinn (1984; 1989), C. Smith (1976), and Tsai (1993: 65–72).

6. There are numerous accounts of the Hong Kong plague and the efforts undertaken by the Hong Kong authorities to combat it. By far the most comprehensive and complete description is that of Elizabeth Sinn (1989: 159–83). In addition, see Severn (1925: 116–27) and Pryor (1975: 61–70). These studies are largely based on governmental reports published in the Hong Kong Government's annual *Hong Kong Legislative Council Sessional Papers* and annual *Blue Book Reports on Bubonic Plague*. See particularly Hong Kong Government, *Hong Kong Legislative Council Sessional Papers*, "Governor's Despatch to the Secretary of State with Reference to the Plague," June 20, 1894.

7. NA, USDS, RG 59, M108, Hunt to Uhl, reel 18, no. 21, June 8, 1894.

8. NA, USDS, RG 59, M101, Seymour to Uhl, reel 12, no. 270, June 6, 1894.

9. Over time, as Europeans living in Hong Kong came to think of plague as a disease endemic to poor Chinese, it only roused concern when it directly threatened them. Edith Blake, wife of the governor of Hong Kong (Henry Blake, governed 1897–1903), remarked in 1901: "I think what caused so much panic this year was that more Europeans were attacked than has ever been the case here before. So long as it is only Chinese who are swept off, the community trouble themselves little about it, but when Europeans get plague, it is considered very terrible" (quoted in Lo 1976: 171).

10. The reason for these differences in case-fatality rates is not clear, but it does not appear to be due to differential medical treatment. Western therapies were not very effective when administered to Chinese victims, as evidenced by the fact that the case-fatality rates of those Chinese who received treatment in foreign clinics were the same as those who did not (see discussion later in this chapter).

11. NA, USDS, RG 59, M101, Seymour to Uhl, reel 12, no. 272, June 27, 1894.

12. Municipal authorities in foreign cities with large Chinese populations used measures consistent with those employed in Hong Kong in 1894. After a dozen cases of bubonic plague were reported in Honolulu in December 1899, 4,500 Chinese were removed to isolation camps and Chinatown was burned down (Trauner 1978: 77). When a dockworker fell ill in Sydney in January 1900, Australian authorities forced Chinese residents of the city to move into tents set up on a local beach (Curson 1985: 152). In March 1900 the San Francisco health officer instructed the chief of police to blockade the entire Chinese district after a 41-year-old Chinese man was determined to have died from plague (McClain 1988: 452; Kraut 1994: 84). Health officials proceeded to conduct house-to-house inspections of all Chinese residences, followed by the fumigation and cleanup of dwellings (McClain 1988: 462). The surgeon general of the Marine Hospital Service (forerunner to the United States Public Health Service) ordered that all Chinese living in San Francisco be inoculated with an experimental vaccine, and preparations were made to remove Chinese residents to detention camps (ibid.: 465). Only the intervention of an enlightened federal judge, who found these measures unconstitutional on the grounds that they were arbitrarily based on race, prevented their being put into effect.

13. NA, USDS, RG 59, M101, Seymour to Uhl, reel 12, no. 272, June 27, 1894.

14. Western therapies that resulted in case-fatality rates over 90 percent are reported for several foreign hospitals in the following document: NA, USDS, RG 59, M101, McWade to Hill, reel 15, no. 113, June 25, 1901.

15. On resistance to plague control measures in India, see Arnold (1988; 1993: 200–30) and Chandavarkar (1992: 229–32). On late-nineteenth-century European responses to intrusive public-health measures, see Richard Evans (1987: 244).

6. CHINESE STATE MEDICINE

1. The Customs Service and the foreign port health officer (generally the customs medical officer) supervised quarantine in the treaty ports. The superintendent of customs declared a city infected, and the medical officer enforced the measure.

2. Temporary stations had been set up in 1894, 1896, and 1898. A permanent station was built in April 1899.

3. See also NA, USDS, RG 59, M105, Gracey to Gridler, reel 9, no. 64, July 3, 1899.

4. Zongli Yamen Archives (Taibei), Xu Yingkui communication, Guangxu 27/9/16 (1901), doc. 02-31-1 (1).

5. This memorial is quoted in a court letter sent to Yuan Shikai from the Grand Council (*Junji chu*), which is quoted in turn in his memorial dated Guangxu 30/12/14 (1904; see Yuan Shikai 1971, 6: 1673–75).

6. NA, USDS, RG 59, M100, A. Johnson to Hill, reel 14, no. 101, May 14, 1901.

7. For histories of new-style police in China, see Stapleton (1993), Wakeman (1991; 1992: 110–12), and Wang Jiajian (1984). On the Japanese influence on New Policies police reform, see Reynolds (1993: 161–78).

8. The duties and functions of the Sanitary Department are listed in an undated document held in the Ministry of the Interior Archives (1907–11, file 1509.138). The responsibilities of the department included: (1) the inspection of food and beverages, (2) cleaning of rivers and streets, (3) supervision of "common people's sanitation" (*pinmin weisheng*), (4) sanitation in factories and public places, (5) infectious disease prevention, (6) vaccinations, (7) ship quarantine, (8) regulation of doctors, (9) inspection of medicine and the pharmaceutical industry, and (10) inspection and regulation of hospitals, medical schools, benevolent halls, and all other institutions involved in health care.

9. There is no doubt that the system was being used in some provinces before the fall of the dynasty. A *Jingwu gongsuo* (Police Daotai) was established in Canton in 1909 along with a sanitary division (*Nanhaixian zhi* 1910, 6: 2b). In Fuzhou, a Police Daotai office was inaugurated in 1909, and a sanitary division was set up two years later, in July 1911 (Inspectorate General, *Decennial Reports* 1902–11, 2: 97). The Longzhou Police Daotai Office was established along with a sanitary division in 1907 (ibid.: 270). By 1911, Police Daotai offices were found in virtually all provinces (Brunnert and Hagelstrom 1912: 421). It is not possible to say, however, how many of these offices had also established sanitary divisions.

10. For a discussion of the development of Chinese state medicine in the Republican era, see AnElissa Lucas (1982). Lucas makes a similar point about the significance of the 1910–11 pneumonic plague epidemic for the development of later state medical systems (ibid.: 45).

11. It is not clear how successful these early efforts at police and sanitation reform in Fengtian province actually were. In his history of police reform in China, Wang Jiajian (1984: 94) enumerates a number of difficulties facing the new-style police department in Fengtian: lack of talented men, abuse of finances, and overall disorganization.

12. On Xiliang and his reform program in the northeast, see Des Forges (1973: 160–79).

13. This estimate is corroborated by a document dated February 25, 1911, archived in the United States State Department Decimal File, which places the number of police officers in Fengtian province at 11,000 and in the city of Shenyang at 4,000. See NA, USDS, RG 59, General Records, Decimal File, Fisher to Calhoun, file no. 158.931/139, Feb. 25, 1911.

14. Zhang Yuanqi, the commissioner of the interior, coordinated the police force and the administrative response to plague in Shenyang. The commissioner of foreign affairs, Han Guojun, coordinated antiplague efforts with the foreign powers. On the international politics of the plague epidemic, see Nathan (1967).

15. These seven districts and the location of each plague prevention station

can be found on the Shenyang city map included in *Fengtian tongzhi* (Gazetteer of Fengtian; 1982 [1934], *juan* 1). See also Leeming (1970).

16. NA, USDS, RG 59, General Records, Decimal File, Fisher to Department of State, file no. 158.931/97, Jan. 17, 1911.

17. Ibid.

18. Ibid.

19. During the months of the epidemic, the *Shengjing shibao* (Mukden times) published daily lists of those who had died of plague, including their names (when known), age, sex, native place, and occupation. By far the majority of those listed were young male coolies from Zhili or Shandong. These workers were generally passing through Shenyang from northern Manchuria, hardest hit by the plague, to their native places.

20. The Shenyang Chamber of Commerce was formed in 1907 as part of the general late-Qing reorganization of merchant associations. It was composed of various *huiguan* that had been active in the city since the eighteenth century. The two most important of these merchant associations were the Shandong and the Zhili guilds, but there were also guilds for sojourners from Shanxi, Jiangxi, Zhejiang, Anhui, Fujian, and Jiangsu. On *huiguan* in Shenyang, see *Chengdexian zhishu* (1967 [1910], 2: 15b).

21. The establishment of the Chamber of Commerce hospital is reported in *Shengjing shibao* Jan. 17, 1911: 5 and also Feb. 16, 1911: 5.

22. Problems with the management of the hospital and its closure are also reported in *Shengjing shibao* Mar. 2, 1911: 5 and Mar. 4, 1911: 5.

23. NA, USDS, RG 59, General Records, Decimal File, Fisher to Department of State, file no. 158.931/152, Feb. 27, 1911.

24. When the Chamber of Commerce announced that it would establish a plague inspection corps of 500 men, it received 5,600 applicants. The stated reason for establishing the corps in the first place was that "those assisting the government [in this task] are insufficient" (*Shengjing shibao* Mar. 2, 1911: 5). Reports on the work of the Chamber of Commerce plague inspection corps are found in ibid. Mar. 29, 1911: 5, Mar. 30, 1911: 5, Apr. 4, 1911: 5, and Apr. 14, 1911: 5. The dispersal of the corps is reported in ibid. Apr. 23, 1911: 5.

WORKS CITED

Works Cited

Works cited in the text and notes by abbreviation are listed, with full bibliographic information, in Abbreviations, pp. xix–xx.

Ackerknecht, Erwin H. 1948. "Anticontagionism Between 1821 and 1867." *Bulletin of the History of Medicine* 22: 562–93.

Adas, Michael. 1989. *Machines as the Measure of Men: Science, Technology, and Ideologies of Western Dominance.* Ithaca, N.Y.: Cornell University Press.

Aijmer, Göran. 1964. *The Dragon Boat Festival on the Hupeh-Hunan Plain: A Study in the Ceremonialism of the Transplantation of Rice.* Stockholm: Ethnographical Museum of Sweden.

Anderson, John. 1972 [1876]. *Mandalay to Momien: A Narrative of the Two Expeditions to Western China of 1868 and 1875 Under Colonel Ed. B. Sladen and Colonel Horace Browne.* Taibei: Chengwen chubanshe.

Anderson, Warwick. 1992. "'Where Every Prospect Pleases and Only Man is Vile': Laboratory Medicine as Colonial Discourse." *Critical Inquiry* 18 (Spring): 506–29.

Anshunfu zhi (Gazetteer of Anshun prefecture). 1851. Chang En (comp.).

Arnold, David. 1988. "Touching the Body: Perspectives on the Indian Plague, 1896–1900." In Ranajit Guha and Gayatri Chakravorty Spivak, eds., *Selected Subaltern Studies,* pp. 391–426. New York: Oxford University Press.

———. 1993. *Colonizing the Body: State Medicine and Epidemic Disease in Nineteenth-Century India.* Berkeley: University of California Press.

Baishansi zhi (Gazetteer of Baishan township). 1830. Wang Yanji (comp.).

Baldwin, Martha. 1993. "Toads and Plague: Amulet Therapy in Seventeenth-Century Medicine." *Bulletin of the History of Medicine* 67, no. 2: 227–47.

Ball, Dyer. 1895. "A Chinese View of Plague." In Hong Kong Government, *Hong Kong Legislative Council Sessional Papers.* Hong Kong: Government Printers.

Beal, Edwin George, Jr. 1958. *The Origin of Likin (1853–1864).* Cambridge, Mass.: Harvard University Press, Chinese Economic and Political Studies.

Beiliuxian zhi (Gazetteer of Beiliu county). 1880. Xu Zuomei (comp.).

Benedict, Carol. 1992. "Bubonic Plague in Nineteenth-Century China." Ph.D. diss., Stanford University.

Benedictow, Ole J. 1987. "Morbidity in Historical Plague Epidemics." *Population Studies* 41: 401–31.

———. 1992. *Plague in the Late Medieval Nordic Countries: Epidemiological Studies.* Oslo: Middelalderforlaget.

Bijiexian zhi (Gazetteer of Bijie county). 1879. Chen Changyan (comp.).

Binyangxian zhi (Gazetteer of Binyang county). 1948. Binyangxian wenxian weiyuanhui (comp.).

Binzhou zhi (Gazetteer of Binzhou department). 1826. Geng Shengxiu (comp.).

Binzhou zhi (Gazetteer of Binzhou department). 1886. Geng Shengxiu (comp.).

Biraben, Jean-Noël. 1975. *Les Hommes et la peste en France et dans les pays européens et méditerranéens.* 2 vols. Paris: Mouton.

Boseting zhi (Gazetteer of Bose subprefecture). 1891. Chen Rujin (comp.).

Bradford, M. G., and W. A. Kent. 1989 [1977]. *Human Geography: Theories and Applications.* Oxford: Oxford University Press.

Brand, Jeanne. 1965. *Doctors and the State.* Baltimore, Md.: Johns Hopkins Press.

Brunnert, H. S., and V. V. Hagelstrom. 1912. *Present Day Political Organization of China.* Trans. A. Beltchenko and E. E. Morgan. Shanghai: Kelly and Walsh.

Carmichael, Ann. 1986. *Plague and the Poor in Renaissance Florence.* Cambridge, Eng.: Cambridge University Press.

———. 1993. "Bubonic Plague." In Kenneth Kiple, ed., *The Cambridge World History of Human Disease*, pp. 628–31. Cambridge, Eng.: Cambridge University Press.

Carné, Louis de. 1982 [1872]. *Travels in Indo-China and the Chinese Empire.* London: Chapman and Hall.

Catanach, I. J. 1983. "Plague and the Indian Village, 1896–1914." In Peter Robb, ed., *Rural India: Land, Power, and Society Under British Rule*, pp. 216–43. London: Curzon Press.

———. 1987. "Poona Politicians and the Plague." In Jim Masselos, ed., *Struggling and Ruling: The Indian National Congress, 1885–1985*, pp. 198–215. London: Oriental University Press.

———. 1988. "Plague and the Tensions of Empire: India, 1896–1918." In David Arnold, ed., *Imperial Medicine and Indigenous Societies*, pp. 149–71. Manchester: Manchester University Press.

Chandavarkar, Rajnaraya. 1992. "Plague Panic and Epidemic Politics in India, 1868–1914." In Terence Ranger and Paul Slack, eds., *Epidemics and Ideas: Essays on the Historical Perception of Pestilence*, pp. 203–40. Cambridge, Eng.: Cambridge University Press.

Chang, Chia-feng. 1993. "Strategies of Dealing with Smallpox in the Early Qing Imperial Family." Paper presented at the Seventh International Conference on the History of Science in East Asia, Tokyo, Japan.

Chao, Wei-pang. 1943. "The Dragon Boat Race in Wuling, Hunan." *Folklore Studies* 2: 1–18.

Chen Shaoxing. 1985 [1979]. *Taiwan di renkou bianqian yu shehui bianqian* (Population and social change in Taiwan). Taibei: Lianjing chuban shiye gongsi.

Chengdexian zhishu (Gazetteer of Chengde). 1967 [1910] Zhang Ziying (comp.).

Chenggongxian zhi (Gazetteer of Chenggong county). 1885. Zhu Ruogong (comp.).

Choa, G. H. 1981. *The Life and Times of Sir Kai Ho Kai*. Hong Kong: Chinese University of Hong Kong.

Chongshanxian zhi (Gazetteer of Chongshan county). 1937. Wu Longhui (comp.).

Christie, Dugald. 1914. *Thirty Years in the Manchu Capital*. New York: McBride and Nast.

Chuxiongxian zhi (Gazetteer of Chuxiong county). 1910. Chong Qian (comp.).

Cliff, A. D., P. Haggett, J. K. Ord, and G. R. Versey. 1981. *Spatial Diffusion: An Historical Geography of Epidemics in an Island Community*. Cambridge, Eng.: Cambridge University Press.

Cohen, Paul. 1984. *Discovering History in China*. New York: Columbia University Press.

Colquhoun, Archibald R. 1883. *Across Chryse*. 2 vols. London: S. Low, Marston, Searle, and Rivington.

Cooper, Thomas T. 1869. "Notes on Western China." *Proceedings of the Asiatic Society of Bengal*. May, pp. 143–55.

———. 1871a. "On the Chinese Province of Yunnan and its Borders." *Proceedings of the Royal Geographical Society* 15 (Mar. 27): 163–74.

———. 1871b. *Travels of a Pioneer of Commerce in Pigtails and Petticoats*. London: J. Murray.

Cousland, Philip. 1896. "The Bubonic Plague in Swatow." *China Medical Missionary Journal* 10, no. 1 (Mar.): 23–24.

Crozier, Ralph. 1968. *Traditional Medicine in Modern China: Science, Nationalism, and the Tensions of Cultural Change*. Cambridge, Mass.: Harvard University Press.

Cunningham, Andrew. 1992. "Transforming Plague: The Laboratory and the Identity of Infectious Disease." In Andrew Cunningham and Perry Williams, eds., *The Laboratory Revolution in Medicine*, pp. 209–44. Cambridge, Eng.: Cambridge University Press.

Curson, Peter. 1985. *Times of Crisis: Epidemics in Sydney, 1788–1900*. Sydney: Sydney University Press.

Cushman, Jennifer. 1975. "Fields from the Sea: Chinese Junk Trade with Siam During the Late Eighteenth and Early Nineteenth Centuries." Ph.D. diss., Cornell University.

Dadingfu zhi (Gazetteer of Dading prefecture). 1849. Huang Zhaizhong (comp.).

Dalixian zhigao (Gazetteer of Dali county). 1917. Zhang Peijue (comp.).

Dataoxian zhi (Gazetteer of Datao county). 1845. Li Xun (comp.).

Deng Tietao. 1955. "Wenbing xueshuo de fazhan yu chengjiu" (The development and accomplishments of the Warm Factor school). *Zhongyi zazhi* (The journal of Chinese medicine) 5: 6–10.

Dengchuanzhou zhi (Gazetteer of Dengchuan department). 1853. Niu Fangtu (comp.).

Des Forges, Roger. 1973. *Hsi-liang and the Chinese National Revolution.* New Haven, Conn.: Yale University Press.

Diamant, Neil. 1992. "Of Asylums, Hospitals, and Prisons: The Transformation of Mental Institutions in China, 1895–1935." Paper presented at the annual meeting of the Association for Asian Studies, Washington, D.C., Apr. 5.

Dianshizhai huabao (Dianshi studio illustrated news). 1983 [1885–95]. Guangzhou: Guangdong renmin chubanshe.

Dikötter, Frank. 1992. *The Discourse of Race in Modern China.* Stanford, Calif.: Stanford University Press.

Dols, Michael W. 1977. *The Black Death in the Middle East.* Princeton, N.J.: Princeton University Press.

Dongfang zazhi (The eastern miscellany). 1904–5. Shanghai: Commercial Press.

Duara, Prasenjit. 1988a. *Culture, Power, and the State: Rural North China, 1900–1942.* Stanford, Calif.: Stanford University Press.

———. 1988b. "Superscribing Symbols: The Myth of Guandi, Chinese God of War." *Journal of Asian Studies* 47, no. 4 (Nov.): 778–95.

———. 1991. "Knowledge and Power in the Discourse of Modernity: The Campaigns Against Popular Religion in Early Twentieth-Century China." *Journal of Asian Studies* 50, no. 1 (Feb.): 67–83.

Duffy, John. 1993. "History of Public Health and Sanitation in the West since 1700." In Kenneth Kiple, ed., *The Cambridge World History of Human Disease,* pp. 200–206. Cambridge, Eng.: Cambridge University Press.

Duke, James A. 1985. *CRC Handbook of Medicinal Herbs.* Boca Raton, Fla.: CRC Press.

Dunstan, Helen. 1975. "The Late Ming Epidemics: A Preliminary Survey." *Ch'ing-shih Wen-t'i* 3, no. 3 (Nov.): 1–59.

Dutton, Michael. 1992. *Policing and Punishment in China.* Hong Kong: Cambridge University Press.

Eckert, Edward. 1978. "Boundary Formation and the Diffusion of Plague: Swiss Epidemics from 1562–1669." *Annales de demographie historique,* pp. 49–80.

———. 1982. "Spatial and Temporal Distribution of Plague in a Region of Switzerland in the Years 1628 and 1629." *Bulletin of the History of Medicine* 56, no. 1: 175–94.

Endacott, G. B. 1958. *A History of Hong Kong.* London: Oxford University Press.

Esherick, Joseph, and Mary Rankin. 1990. *Chinese Local Elites and Patterns of Dominance.* Berkeley: University of California Press.

Evans, Richard J. 1987. *Death in Hamburg: Society and Politics in the Cholera Years, 1830–1910.* London: Viking, Penguin.

Fan Xingzhun. 1986. *Zhongguo yixue shilue* (A brief history of Chinese medicine). Beijing: Zhongyi guji chubanshe.

Fang Yaozhong and Xu Jiasong. 1986. *Wenbing huijiang* (Compilation on Warm Factor disorders). Beijing: Renmin weisheng chubanshe.

Farquhar, Judith. 1994. *Knowing Practice: The Clinical Encounter of Chinese Medicine.* Boulder, Colo.: Westview.

Farquhar, Judith, and James Hevia. 1993. "Culture and Postwar American Historiography of China." *Positions: East Asia Cultures Critique* 1, no. 2 (Fall): 486–525.

Fee, Elizabeth, and Dorothy Porter. 1992. "Public Health, Preventive Medicine and Professionalization: England and America in the Nineteenth Century." In Andrew Wear, ed., *Medicine in Society: Historical Essays,* pp. 249–75. Cambridge, Eng.: Cambridge University Press.

Fengtian tongzhi (Comprehensive gazetteer of Fengtian province). 1982 [1934]. Zhai Wenxuan (comp.).

Fenton, James. 1994. "The Disease of All Diseases." *The New York Review of Books.* Dec. 1, p. 48.

Forbes, Andrew. 1987. "The 'CinHo' (Yunnanese Chinese) Caravan Trade with Northern Thailand During the Late Nineteenth and Early Twentieth Centuries." *Journal of Asian History,* pp. 1–47.

Foster, Burnside. 1894. "The Bubo Plague in China." *Journal of the American Medical Association.* Sept. 22, p. 7.

Fu Weikang. 1984. "Wo guo jindai fangyishi shang de jiechu zhanshi—Wu Liande" (Wu Lien-teh—An outstanding fighter in our country's modern epidemic control history). *Zhongguo keji shiliao* (Historical materials on China's science and technology) 5, no. 4: 64–66.

Gao Hesheng. 1979. "Cong Wu Youke, Ye Tianshi, Wu Jutong, san jia xueshuo kan wenbingxue de fazhan" (The development of the Warm Factor school viewed from the theories of Wu Youke, Ye Tianshi, and Wu Jutong). *Zhejiang zhongyiyao* (Zhejiang journal of Chinese medicine) 7: 225–28.

Gill, William R. E. 1883. *The River of Golden Sand: Being the Narrative of a Journey Through China and Eastern Tibet to Burma.* London: John Murray.

Gong Chun. 1959. "Mingdai de weisheng zuzhi yu yixue jiaoyu" (The health system and medical education of the Ming dynasty). *Renmin baojian* (The people's health) 7: 680–84.

———. 1960. "Qingdai de yishi zhidu shiliao" (Historical materials on the Qing dynasty's medical system). *Renmin baojian* (The people's health) 4: 223–25.

Gongzhongdang Guangxuchao zouzhe (Secret palace memorials of the Guangxu period, 1875–1908). 1973–75. Vol. 8. Taibei: National Palace Museum.

Goodrich, Anne. 1964. *The Peking Temple of the Eastern Peak: The Tung-yueh Miao in Peking and its Lore.* Nagoya, Japan: Monumenta Serica.

Gottfried, Robert S. 1983. *The Black Death.* New York: Free Press.

Gou Qianheng. 1985. "Wenbingxue fazhan shilue" (A brief history of the development of the Warm Factor school). *Zhonghua yishi zazhi* (Journal of Chinese medical history) 15, no. 2 (Apr.): 84–88.

Government-General of Taiwan (Taiwan Sōtokufu), Office of Police Affairs (Keimu Kyoku), Public Health Section (Eiseika). 1924. *Eisei chōsa sho* (Report on the investigation of public health). Taihoku (Taibei).

Grandstaff, T. B. 1979. "The Hmong, Opium and the Haw: Speculations on the

Origins of Their Association." *Journal of the Siam Society* 67, no. 2 (July): 70–79.

Guangdong tongzhi (Comprehensive gazetteer of Guangdong province). 1864. Chen Changqi (comp.).

Guixian zhi (Gazetteer of Guixian county). 1935. Ou Yangxi (comp.).

Guizhousheng tushuguan (Guizhou Provincial Library). 1982. *Guizhou lidai ziran huohai nianbiao* (A chronological table of natural disasters in Guizhou's history). Guiyang: Guizhou renmin chubanshe.

Hägerstrand, Torsten. 1967 [1953]. *Innovation Diffusion as a Spatial Process*. Trans. A. Pred. Chicago: University of Chicago Press.

Hanson, Marta. 1991. "External Chaos, Internal Disorder: Chinese Medical Concepts of Epidemics." Paper presented at the annual meeting of the Association for Asian Studies, New Orleans, Apr. 11–14.

———. Forthcoming. "External Chaos, Internal Disorder: The Creation of a Southern Medical Tradition on Heat Factor Disorders During the Qing Dynasty." Ph.D. diss., University of Pennsylvania.

Hayes, James. 1977. *The Hong Kong Region, 1850–1911: Institutions and Leadership in Town and Countryside*. Hamden, Conn.: Archon Books, The Shoe String Press.

———. 1983. *The Rural Communities of Hong Kong: Studies and Themes*. Hong Kong: Oxford University Press.

He Bin. 1988. "Wo guo nueji liuxing jianshi" (A brief history of the spread of malaria in China). *Zhonghua yishi zazhi* (Journal of Chinese medical history) 18, no. 1: 1–8.

He Changling. 1886. *Huangchao jingshi wenbian* (Collected writings on statecraft of the reigning dynasty). Wujin sibu lou.

Hechizhou zhi (Gazetteer of Hechi department). 1907. Li Youyuan (comp.).

Heqingxian zhi (Gazetteer of Heqing county). 1923. Yang Jinkai (comp.).

Heqingzhou zhi (Gazetteer of Heqing department). 1894. Wang Baoyi (comp.).

Herzlich, Claudine, and Janine Pierret. 1987. *Illness and Self in Society*. Baltimore, Md.: Johns Hopkins University Press.

Hill, Ann Maxwell. 1989. "Chinese Dominance of the Xishuangbanna Tea Trade." *Modern China* 15, no. 3: 321–45.

Hirst, L. Fabian. 1953. *The Conquest of Plague: A Study of the Evolution of Epidemiology*. Oxford: Clarendon Press.

Hirth, Friedrich, and W. W. Rockhill. 1911. *Chau Ju-kua: His Work on the Chinese and Arab Trade in the Twelfth and Thirteenth Centuries, Entitled "Chu-fan-chi."* St. Petersburg: Imperial Academy of Sciences.

Hong Kong Government. 1894–1907. *Blue Book Reports on Bubonic Plague*. Hong Kong: Hong Kong Government Printers.

———. 1894–1908. *Hong Kong Legislative Council Sessional Papers*. Hong Kong: Hong Kong Government Printers.

———. 1932. *Historical and Statistical Abstract of the Colony, 1841–1930*. Hong Kong: Hong Kong Government Printers.

Hong Liangji (Hong Beijiang). 1877–79. *Hong Beijiang xiansheng yiji* (The collected works of Hong Beijiang). Hubei: Shoujingtang.

Hosie, Alexander. 1890. *Three Years in Western China: A Narrative of Three Journeys in Ssu-ch'uan, Kuei-chow, and Yun-nan*. London: George Philip.

Hsu, Francis. 1952. *Religion, Science, and Human Crises: A Study of China in Transition and Its Implications for the West*. London: Routledge and Kegan Paul.

Huang Liu-hung. 1984. *A Complete Book Concerning Happiness and Benevolence*. Trans. Djang Chu. Tucson: University of Arizona Press.

Huang Zhongxian. 1909. *Shuyi fei yi—liu jing tiaobian* (Plague is not an epidemic—Systematic manifestation type-determination in the Six Warps). Guangzhou: Zhenghetang.

Hull, Terence. 1987. "Plague in Java." In Norman Owen, ed., *Death and Disease in Southeast Asia*, pp. 210–34. Singapore: Oxford University Press.

Ichiko, Chūzō. 1980. "Political and Institutional Reform, 1901–11." In John K. Fairbank and Kwang-ching Liu, eds., *The Cambridge History of China*, vol. 11, part 2, pp. 375–415. Cambridge, Eng.: Cambridge University Press.

Iijima, Wataru. 1991. "On the Prevalence of the Plague in Modern East Asia: Guangdong and Xianggang in 1894, Yokohama in 1902–03, and 'Man zhou' in 1910–11." *Shichō* (The journal of history) 29 (June): 24–39.

"Infection in Bubonic Plague." 1896. *China Medical Missionary Journal* 5, no. 1 (Mar.): 54.

Inspectorate General of Chinese Imperial Customs. Special Series, II, *Customs Medical Reports*. Nos. 14–16 (1877–78); 24 (1882); 33–39 (1887–90); 40–50 (1890–95); 58–64 (1899–1902); 68–80 (1904–10). Shanghai: Statistical Department of the Inspectorate General of Customs.

Inspectorate General of Chinese Imperial Customs. *Decennial Reports 1882–91, 1892–1901, 1902–11*. Shanghai: Statistical Department of the Inspectorate General of Customs.

International Plague Conference. 1912. *Report of the International Plague Conference, Mukden, 1911*. Manila: Bureau of Printing.

Janetta, Ann. 1987. *Epidemics and Mortality in Early Modern Japan*. Princeton, N.J.: Princeton University Press.

Jen, Yu-wen. 1973. *The Taiping Revolutionary Movement*. New Haven, Conn.: Yale University Press.

Ji Shuli. 1988. *Shuyi* (Plague). Beijing: Renmin weisheng chubanshe.

Jingdong zhiliting zhi (Gazetteer of Jingdong autonomous subprefecture). 1788. Wu Lansong (comp.).

Jingdongfu zhi (Gazetteer of Jingdong prefecture). 1732. Xu Shuhong (comp.).

Jingdongxian zhigao (Gazetteer of Jingdong county). 1923. Zhou Ruzhao (comp.).

Johnston, William. 1987. "Disease, Medicine, and the State: A Social History of Tuberculosis in Japan, 1850–1950." Ph.D. diss., Harvard University.

Katz, Paul. 1987. "Demons or Deities—The Wangye of Taiwan." *Asian Folklore Studies* 46: 197–215.

———. 1990. "Plague Festivals in Chekiang in Late Imperial China." Ph.D. diss., Princeton University.

————. 1991. "Religious Responses to Epidemics in Late Imperial China." Paper presented at the annual meeting of the Association for Asian Studies, New Orleans, Apr. 11–14.

Kerr, John. 1894. "The Bubonic Plague." *The China Medical Missionary Journal* 13, no. 4 (Dec.): 178–80.

Klein, Ira. 1986. "Urban Development and Death: Bombay City, 1870–1914." *Modern Asian Studies* 20, no. 4: 725–54.

————. 1988. "Plague, Policy and Popular Unrest in British India." *Modern Asian Studies* 22, no. 4: 723–55.

Kraut, Alan. 1994. *Silent Travelers: Germs, Genes, and the "Immigrant Menace."* New York: Basic Books.

Kunmingxian zhi (Gazetteer of Kunming county). 1901 [1841]. Dai Jiongsun (comp.).

Kunmingxian zhi (Gazetteer of Kunming county). 1939. Ni Weiqin (comp.).

Kuriyama, Shigehisa. 1993. "Concepts of Disease in East Asia." In Kenneth Kiple, ed., *The Cambridge World History of Human Disease*, pp. 52–59. Cambridge, Eng.: Cambridge University Press.

————. 1994. "The Imagination of Winds and the Development of the Chinese Conception of the Body." In Angela Zito and Tani E. Barlow, eds., *Body, Subject, and Power in China*, pp. 23–41. Chicago: University of Chicago Press.

Laai, Yi-faai. 1950. "The Part Played by the Pirates of Kwangtung and Kwangsi Provinces in the Taiping Insurrection." Ph.D. diss., University of California, Berkeley.

Laai, Yi-faai, Franz Michael, and John C. Sherman. 1962. "The Use of Maps in Social Research: A Case Study in South China." *Geographical Review* 52: 92–111.

Laffey, Ella S. 1972. "The Making of a Rebel: Liu Yung-fu and the Formation of the Black Flag Army." In Jean Chesneaux, ed., *Popular Movements and Secret Societies in China, 1840–1950*, pp. 85–96. Stanford, Calif.: Stanford University Press.

————. 1975. "French Adventurers and Chinese Bandits in Tonkin: The Garnier Affair in Its Local Context." *Journal of Southeast Asian Studies* 6, no. 1: 38–51.

————. 1976. "In the Wake of the Taipings: Some Patterns of Local Revolt in Kwangsi Province, 1850–1875." *Modern Asian Studies* 10, no. 1: 65–81.

Lang, Graeme, and Lars Ragvald. 1993. *The Rise of a Refugee God: Hong Kong's Wong Tai Sin.* Hong Kong: Oxford University Press.

Langqiongxian zhilue (Records of Langqiong county). 1903. Zhou Hang (comp.).

Lao Tong. 1935–40 [1794]. "Jiuhuang beilan" (Materials for famine administration). In Wang Yunwu (comp.), *Congshu jicheng* (Collected collectanea). Shanghai: Commercial Press.

Lary, Diana. 1974. *Region and Nation: The Kwangsi Clique in Chinese Politics, 1925–1937.* London: Cambridge University Press.

Lee, James. 1982a. "Food Supply and Population Growth in Southwest China, 1250–1850." *Journal of Asian Studies* 41, no. 4 (Aug.): 711–801.

————. 1982b. "The Legacy of Immigration in Southwest China, 1250–1850." *Annales de démographie historique* 1: 279–304.

————. 1993. "State and Economy in Southwest China, 1250–1850." Unpublished manuscript.

Lee, Robert. 1979. "Frontier Politics in the Southwestern Sino-Tibetan Borderlands During the Ch'ing Dynasty." In Joshua Fogel and William Rowe, eds., *Perspectives on a Changing China*, pp. 35–68. Boulder, Colo.: Westview Press.

Lee, T'ao. 1958. "Chinese Medicine During the Ming Dynasty." *Chinese Medical Journal* 76 (Feb.–Mar.): 178–98, 285–304.

Leeming, Frank. 1970. "Reconstructing Late Ch'ing Feng-t'ien." *Modern Asian Studies* 4, no. 4: 305–24.

————. 1977. *Street Studies in Hong Kong: Localities in a Chinese City.* Hong Kong: Oxford University Press.

Lethbridge, Henry. 1978. *Hong Kong: Stability and Change.* Hong Kong: Oxford University Press.

Leung, Angela. 1987. "Organized Medicine in Ming-Qing China: State and Private Medical Institutions in the Lower Yangzi Region." *Late Imperial China* 8, no. 1: 134–66.

Li Hanzhang. 1967 [1900] *Hefei Li Jinke gong (Hanzhang) zhengshu* (The political correspondence of Li Jinke [Hanzhang]). Li Jingyu (comp.). 2 vols. Taibei: Wenhai chubanshe.

Li Yaonan. 1954. "Yunnan zhangqi (nueji) liuxing jianshi" (A short history of endemic malaria in Yunnan). *Zhonghua yishi zazhi* (Journal of Chinese medical history) 3: 180–83.

Lianzhoufu zhi (Gazetteer of Lianzhou prefecture). 1833. Zhang Yuchun (comp.).

Liao Tingxiang. 1967 [1889]. *Guangdong yudi quanshou* (Complete explication of the atlas of Guangdong province). Taibei: Chengwen chubanshe.

Lijiangfu zhi (Gazetteer of Lijiang prefecture). 1895. Chen Zonghai (comp.).

Lin Manhong. 1985. "Qingmo shehui liudong xishi yapian yanjiu—gonggei mian zhi fenxi" (A supply side analysis of the prevalence of opium-smoking in late Ch'ing China, 1773–1906). Ph.D. diss., National Taiwan Normal University.

Lin Shiquan. 1989. "Hainan dao beibuqu shuyi liuxing shiliao" (Historical materials on the spread of plague in northern Hainan Island). *Zhonghua yishi zazhi* (Journal of Chinese medical history) 19, no. 2 (Apr.): 100–101.

Ling, L. C., K. B. Liu, and Y. T. Yao. 1936. "Studies on the So-called Chang-ch'i: Chang-ch'i in Yunnan." *Chinese Medical Journal* 50 (Dec.): 1815–28.

Linguixian zhi (Gazetteer of Lingui county). 1905. Wu Zheng'ao (comp.).

Liu Zhiwan. 1962. "The Belief and Practice of the *Wenshen* Cult in South China and Formosa." In *Proceedings of the Second Biennial Conference*, pp. 715–22. Taibei: International Association of Historians of Asia.

————. 1966. "The Temple of the Gods of Epidemics in Taiwan." *Academica Sinica Bulletin of the Institute of Ethnology* 22: 53–95.

————. 1983. *Taiwan minjian xinyang lunji* (Collected essays on Taiwanese popular beliefs). Taibei: Lianjing chuban shiye.

Liujiangxian zhi (Gazetteer of Liujiang county). 1937. Xiao Dianyuan (comp.).

Lo, Hui-min. 1976. *The Correspondence of G. E. Morrison, 1895–1912.* 2 vols. Cambridge, Eng.: Cambridge University Press.

Lombard-Salmon, Claudine. 1972. *Un exemple d'acculturation Chinoise: La province du Gui Zhou au XVIIIe siècle.* Paris: Ecole Française d'Extrême-Orient.

Longanxian zhi (Gazetteer of Longan county). 1934. Liu Zhenxi (comp.).

Longzhou jilue (Records of Longzhou). 1803. Huang Yu (comp.).

Lucas, AnElissa. 1982. *Chinese Medical Modernization: Comparative Policy Continuities, 1930–1980s.* New York: Praeger.

Luliangxian zhigao (Gazetteer of Luliang county). 1915. Liu Runchou (comp.).

Lum, Raymond D. 1985. "Philanthropy and Public Welfare in Late Imperial China." Ph.D. diss., Harvard University.

Luopingxian zhi (Gazetteer of Luoping county). 1933. Zhu Wei (comp.).

Luoyuanxian weiyuan hui. 1985. *Luoyuan wenshi ziliao* (Historical records of Luoyuan). Luoyuan county, Fujian: Luoyuanxian yinshuachang.

Luquanxian zhi (Gazetteer of Luquan county). 1928. Quan Huanze (comp.).

McClain, Charles. 1988. "Of Medicine, Race, and American Law: The Bubonic Plague Outbreak of 1900." *Law and Social Inquiry* 13 (Summer): 447–513.

McNeill, William. 1976. *Plagues and Peoples.* Garden City, N.J.: Anchor Press, Doubleday.

Maguanxian zhi (Gazetteer of Maguan county). 1932. Zhang Ziming (comp.).

Mann, Susan. 1987. *Local Merchants and the Chinese Bureaucracy, 1750–1950.* Stanford, Calif.: Stanford University Press.

Menghua xianxiang tuzhi (Gazetteer of Menghua county). N.d. Guangxu edition. Liang Youyi (comp.).

Menghua zhigao (Gazetteer of Menghua). 1920. Li Chuxi (comp.).

Mengzixian zhi (Gazetteer of Mengzi county). 1797 [1791]. Li Kun (comp.).

Metzgar, Harold D. 1973. "Foreign Penetration and the Rise of Nationalism in Yunnan, 1895–1903." Ph.D. diss., Harvard University.

Metzger, Thomas. 1973. *The Internal Organization of the Ch'ing Bureaucracy: Legal, Normative, and Communication Aspects.* Cambridge, Mass.: Harvard University Press.

Mianningxian zhi (Gazetteer of Mianning county). 1945. Qiu Yanhe (comp.).

Ministry of the Interior Archives. 1907–11. Number One Historical Archives, Beijing. File 1509.138.

Murray, Dian. 1987. *Pirates of the South China Coast, 1790–1810.* Stanford, Calif.: Stanford University Press.

Nanhaixian zhi (Gazetteer of Nanhai county). 1910. Zhang Fengjie (comp.).

Nanningfu zhi (Gazetteer of Nanning prefecture). 1847. Su Shijun (comp.).

Naquin, Susan, and Evelyn Rawski. 1987. *Chinese Society in the Eighteenth Century.* New Haven, Conn.: Yale University Press.

Nathan, Carl. 1967. *Plague Prevention and Politics in Manchuria, 1910–1931.* Cambridge, Mass.: East Asian Research Center, Harvard University.

New York Times. 1994.

Niles, Mary. 1894. "Plague in Canton." *China Medical Missionary Journal* 8, no. 2 (June): 116–19.

Norris, John. 1977. "East or West? The Geographic Origin of the Black Death." *Bulletin of the History of Medicine* 51, no. 1 (Spring): 1–24.

Nutton, Vivan. 1983. "The Seeds of Disease: An Explanation of Contagion and Infection from the Greeks to the Renaissance." *Medical History* 27: 1–34.

Ortholan, Dr. 1908. "La Pest en Indo-Chine (Historique)." *Annales d'hygiène et de médecine coloniales* 11, no. 2 (Avril–Juin): 633–38.

Panyuxian xu zhi (Gazetteer of Panyu county). 1931. Liang Dingfen (comp.).

Park, Katharine. 1993. "Black Death." In Kenneth Kiple, ed., *The Cambridge World History of Human Disease*, pp. 612–16. Cambridge, Eng.: Cambridge University Press.

Pinglefu zhi (Gazetteer of Pingle prefecture). 1805. Qing Gui (comp.).

Pollitzer, R. 1954. *Plague*. Geneva: World Health Organization.

Pollitzer, R., and Karl Meyer. 1961. "The Ecology of Plague." In Jacques May, ed., *Studies in Disease Ecology*, pp. 433–501. New York: Hafner.

Prasertkul, Chiranan. 1989. *Yunnan Trade in the Nineteenth Century: Southwest China's Cross-Boundaries Functional System*. Bangkok: Institute of Asian Studies, Chulalongkorn University.

Provincial Government of Taiwan, Bureau of Accounting and Statistics. 1946. *Taiwan sheng wushiyinian lai de tongji yaolan* (Statistical summary of Taiwan province over the past fifty-one years). Taibei: Bureau of Accounting and Statistics.

Pryor, E. G. 1975. "The Great Plague of Hong Kong." *Journal of the Hong Kong Branch of the Royal Asiatic Society* 15: 61–70.

Pu'erfu zhi (Gazetteer of Pu'er prefecture). 1850 [1840]. Zheng Shaojian (comp.).

Pu'erfu zhigao (Gazetteer of Pu'er prefecture). 1900. Chen Zonghai (comp.).

Pyle, Gerald F. 1969. "The Diffusion of Cholera in the United States in the Nineteenth Century." *Geographical Analysis* 1: 59–75.

———. 1979. *Applied Medical Geography*. Washington, D.C.: V. H. Winston.

———. 1986. *The Diffusion of Influenza: Patterns and Paradigms*. Totowa, N.J.: Rowman and Littlefield.

Qianjiangxian zhi (Gazetteer of Qianjiang county). 1935. Li Xiangpin (comp.).

Qing shi liechuan (Collected biographies of the Qing period). 1962. Taibei: Zhonghua shuju.

Qingyuanfu zhi (Gazetteer of Qingyuan prefecture). 1829. Ying Xiu (comp.).

Qiubeixian zhi (Gazetteer of Qiubei county). 1926. Xu Xiaoxi (comp.).

Rankin, Mary Backus. 1986. *Elite Activism and Political Transformation in China: Zhejiang Province, 1865–1911*. Stanford, Calif.: Stanford University Press.

Reynolds, Douglas. 1993. *China, 1898–1912: The Xinzheng Revolution and Japan*. Cambridge, Mass.: Council on East Asian Studies, Harvard University.

Rhoads, Edward. 1974. "Merchant Associations in Canton, 1895–1911." In Mark Elvin and G. William Skinner, eds., *The Chinese City Between Two Worlds*, pp. 97–117. Stanford, Calif.: Stanford University Press.

Risse, Guenter B. 1992. "'A Long Pull, A Strong Pull, and All Together': San Francisco and the Bubonic Plague, 1907–1908." *Bulletin of the History of Medicine* 66, no. 2 (Summer): 260–86.

Rocher, Emile. 1879. *La province Chinoise du Yunnan*. 2 vols. Paris: Lerous.

Rongxian zhi (Gazetteer of Rong county). 1897. Yi Shaode (comp.).

Rosen, George. 1974. *From Medical Police to Social Medicine: Essays on the History of Health Care.* New York: Neale Watson Academic Publications.

Rosenberg, Charles. 1992. "Introduction: Framing Disease: Illness, Society, and History." In Charles E. Rosenberg and Janet Golden, eds., *Framing Disease: Studies in Cultural History*, pp. xiii–xxvi. New Brunswick, N.J.: Rutgers University Press.

Rowe, William T. 1989. *Hankow: Conflict and Community in a Chinese City, 1796–1895.* Stanford, Calif.: Stanford University Press.

Royal Asiatic Society. 1893–94. "The Inland Communications of China." *Journal of the China Branch of the Royal Asiatic Society* 28: 1–213.

Schipper, Kristofer M. 1985. "Seigneurs royaux, dieux des épidémies" (Royal lords, epidemic gods). *Archives de sciences sociales des religions* 59: 31–40.

Severn, Millott. 1925. "An Outline of the History of Plague in Hong Kong." *The Caduceus: Journal of the Hong Kong University Medical Society* 5, no. 2: 116–27.

Shanglinxian zhi (Gazetteer of Shanglin county). 1899 [1876]. Xu Hengshen (comp.).

Shengjing shibao (Mukden times). 1911.

Shi Changyong. 1957. "Shilun chuanranbing xuejia Wu Youke ji qi 'li qi' xueshuo" (A preliminary discussion of the scholar of infectious disease, Wu Youke, and his theory of *li qi*). *Yixueshi yu baojian zazhi* (Journal of the history of medicine and public health) 9, no. 3: 180–86.

Shi Fan. 1891a. "Ru Dian lucheng kao" (An investigation of the overland roads into Yunnan). In Wang Xiqi, ed., *Xiaofanghu zhai yudi congchao* (Geographical series of Xiaofanghu studio), vol. 11, pp. 6049–53.

———. 1891b. "Ru Mian lucheng" (The road to Burma). In Wang Xiqi, ed., *Xiaofanghu zhai yudi congchao* (Geographical series of Xiaofanghu studio), vol. 13, pp. 7913–14.

Shi Yiren. 1955. "Wenbing fazhan jianshi" (A brief history of the development of the Warm Factor school). *Zhonghua yishi zazhi* (Journal of Chinese medical history) 4: 259–62.

Shichengxian zhi (Gazetteer of Shicheng county). 1892. Jiang Yangui (comp.).

Shichengxian zhi (Gazetteer of Shicheng county). 1931. Zhong Xizhuo (comp.).

Shipingxian zhi (Gazetteer of Shiping county). 1938. Yuan Jiagu (comp.).

Shrewsbury, J. F. D. 1970. *A History of Bubonic Plague in the British Isles.* Cambridge, Eng.: Cambridge University Press.

Shundexian zhi (Gazetteer of Shunde county). 1929. Zhou Zhizhen (comp.).

Simpson, William. 1905. *A Treatise on Plague.* Cambridge, Eng.: Cambridge University Press.

Sinanfu xu zhi (Gazetteer of Sinan prefecture). 1841. Xia Xiunu (comp.).

Sinn, Elizabeth. 1984. "Materials for Historical Research: The Case of a Historical Institution." In Alan Birch, Y. C. Jao, and Elizabeth Sinn, eds., *Research Materials for Hong Kong Studies*, pp. 195–233. Hong Kong: University of Hong Kong, Centre of Asian Studies.

———. 1989. *Power and Charity: The Early History of the Tung Wah Hospital.* Hong Kong: Oxford University Press.

Sivin, Nathan. 1987. *Traditional Medicine in Contemporary China*. Ann Arbor: University of Michigan Center for Chinese Studies.

———. 1993. "Huang-ti nei-ching." In Michael Loewe, ed., *Early Chinese Texts: A Bibliographical Guide*. Berkeley: Institute of East Asian Studies, University of California.

Skinner, G. William. 1957. *Chinese Society in Thailand: An Analytical History*. Ithaca, N.Y.: Cornell University Press.

———. 1977a. "Cities and the Hierarchy of Local Systems." In G. William Skinner, ed., *The City in Late Imperial China*, pp. 275–364. Stanford, Calif.: Stanford University Press.

———. 1977b. "Regional Urbanization in Nineteenth-Century China." In G. William Skinner, ed., *The City in Late Imperial China*, pp. 211–49. Stanford, Calif.: Stanford University Press.

———. 1985. "The Structure of Chinese History." *Journal of Asian Studies* 44, no. 2: 271–92.

Slack, Paul. 1985. *The Impact of Plague in Tudor and Stuart England*. London: Routledge and Kegan Paul.

———. 1988. "Responses to Plague in Early Modern Europe: The Implications of Public Health." *Social Research* 55, no. 3 (Autumn): 433–53.

———. 1992. "Introduction." In Terence Ranger and Paul Slack, eds., *Epidemics and Ideas: Essays on Historical Perception of Pestilence*. Cambridge, Eng.: Cambridge University Press.

Smith, Carl. 1976. "Visit to the Tung Wah Group of Hospitals' Museum, 2nd October, 1976." *Journal of the Hong Kong Branch of the Royal Asiatic Society* 16: 262–80.

Smith, Porter F. 1969. *Chinese Materia Medica: Vegetable Kingdom*. Taibei: Ku T'ing Book House.

Sontag, Susan. 1988. "AIDS and Its Metaphors." *The New York Review of Books*. Oct. 27, pp. 89–99.

Spence, Jonathan. 1975. "Opium Smoking in Ch'ing China." In Frederic Wakeman Jr. and Carolyn Grant, eds., *Conflict and Control in Late Imperial China*, pp. 143–73. Berkeley: University of California Press.

Stapleton, Kristin. 1993. "Police Reform in a Late-Imperial Chinese City: Chengdu, 1902–1911." Ph.D. diss., Harvard University.

Stock, Robert F. 1976. *Cholera in Africa: Diffusion of the Disease, 1970–1975, with Particular Emphasis on West Africa*. London: International African Institute.

Suiyangxian zhi (Gazetteer of Suiyang county). 1928. Hu Ren (comp.).

Sun, E-Tu Zen. 1968. "The Ch'ing Government and the Mineral Industries Before 1800." *Journal of Asian Studies* 25, no. 3 (Aug.): 835–45.

———. 1971. "The Transportation of Yunnan Copper to Peking in the Ch'ing period." *Journal of Oriental Studies* 9: 132–48.

Sung, Kwang-Yu. 1990. "Religion and Society in Ch'ing and Japanese Colonial Taipei." Ph.D. diss., University of Pennsylvania.

Swanson, Maynard. 1977. "The Sanitation Syndrome: Bubonic Plague and Urban Native Policy in the Cape Colony, 1900–1909." *Journal of African History* 18, no. 3: 387–410.

Taiwan sheng tongzhigao (Gazetteer of Taiwan province). 1951–1960. Taiwan wenxian weiyuanhui (comp.). Taibei: Chengwen chubanshe youxian gongsi.

Tan Qixiang. 1980. *Zhongguo lishi ditu ji* (The historical atlas of China). Vol. 8. Beijing: Ditu chubanshe.

Tengyuezhou zhi (Gazetteer of Tengyue subprefecture). 1790. Tu Shulian (comp.).

Tian Jingguo. 1987. *Yunnan yiyao weisheng jian shi* (A concise history of medicine in Yunnan). Kunming: Keji chubanshe.

T'ien, Ju-k'ang. 1982. "New Light on the Yunnan Rebellion and the Panthay Mission." *Memoirs of the Research Department of the Tōyō Bunko* 40: 19–56.

Tōa Dōbunkai. 1919. *Shina shōbetsu zenshi* (A gazetteer of all provinces of China). 18 vols. Tokyo.

Trauner, Joan. 1978. "The Chinese as Medical Scapegoats in San Francisco, 1870–1905." *California History* (Spring) 57: 70–87.

Tsai, Jung-fang. 1993. *Hong Kong in Chinese History: Community and Social Unrest in the British Colony, 1842–1913*. New York: Columbia University Press.

Tung Wah Group of Hospitals, Editorial Board. 1961. *Development of the Tung Wah Hospitals, 1870–1960*. Hong Kong: Tong Nam.

Twigg, Graham. 1984. *The Black Death: A Biological Reappraisal*. New York: Schocken Books.

Twitchett, Denis. 1979. "Population and Pestilence in T'ang China." In Wolfgang Bauer, ed., *Studia Sino-Mongolica (Festschrift für Herbert Franke)*, pp. 35–68. Wiesbaden: Franz Steiner Verlag.

Unschuld, Paul. 1985. *Medicine in China: A History of Ideas*. Berkeley: University of California Press.

Velimirovic, B. 1972. "Plague in Southeast Asia: A Brief Historical Summary and Present Geographical Distribution." *Transactions of the Royal Society of Tropical Medicine and Hygiene* 66, no. 3: 479–504.

Wakeman, Frederic. 1966. *Strangers at the Gate: Social Disorder in South China, 1839–1861*. Berkeley: University of California Press.

———. 1972. "The Secret Societies of Kwangtung, 1800–1950." In Jean Chesneaux, ed., *Popular Movements and Secret Societies in China, 1840–1950*, pp. 29–47. Stanford, Calif.: Stanford University Press.

———. 1991. "Models of Historical Change: The Chinese State and Society, 1839–1989." In Kenneth Lieberthal, Joyce Kallgren, Roderick MacFarquhar, and Frederic Wakeman, eds., *Perspectives on Modern China: Four Anniversaries*, pp. 68–101. Armonk, N.J.: M. E. Sharpe.

———. 1992. "American Police Advisers and the Nationalist Chinese Secret Service, 1930–1937." *Modern China* 18, no. 2 (Apr.): 107–37.

Wang Jiajian. 1984. *Qingmou minchu wo guo jingcha xiandaihua de licheng (1901–1928)* (The modernization of the Chinese police system in the late Qing and early Republican periods, 1901–1928). Taibei: Taiwan shangwu yinshu guan.

Wang Xuhuai. 1968. *Xiantong Yunnan huimin shibian* (The Muslim Rebellion during the Xianfeng and Tongzhi reigns). Taibei: Academia Sinica.

Washington Post. 1994.

Wei, Alice Bihyun Gan. 1974. "The Moslem Rebellion in Yunnan: 1855–1873." Ph.D. diss., University of Chicago.

Will, Pierre-Etienne. 1990. *Bureaucracy and Famine in Eighteenth-Century China.* Trans. Elborg Forster. Stanford, Calif.: Stanford University Press.

Will, Pierre-Etienne, and R. Bin Wong. 1991. *Nourish the People: The State Civilian Granary System in China, 1650–1850.* Ann Arbor: Center for Chinese Studies, University of Michigan.

Wong, Chimin K., and Wu Lien-teh. 1935. *History of Chinese Medicine.* Tientsin: The Tientsin Press.

Wright, Mary Clabaugh. 1957. *The Last Stand of Chinese Conservatism: The T'ung-chih Restoration, 1862–1874.* Stanford, Calif.: Stanford University Press.

———. 1968. "Introduction: The Rising Tide of Change." In Mary Clabaugh Wright, ed., *China in Revolution: The First Phase, 1900–1913,* pp. 1–63. New Haven, Conn.: Yale University Press.

Wu, Lien-teh. 1926. *A Treatise on Pneumonic Plague.* Geneva: League of Nations.

———. 1936. *Plague: A Manual for Medical and Public Health Workers.* Shanghai: National Quarantine Service.

———. 1959. *Plague Fighter: The Autobiography of a Modern Chinese Physician.* Cambridge, Eng.: Heffer.

Wuchuanxian zhi (Gazetteer of Wuchuan county). 1892 [1888]. Mao Changshan (comp.).

Wuyuanxian zhi (Gazetteer of Wuyuan county). 1914. Tang Zhaosheng (comp.).

Xia Yihuang. 1935. "Sangjia jiu xi zhi yuyi guan" (Observations on funeral customs to prevent epidemics). *Zhongxi yiyao* (Journal of Chinese and Western medicine) 4 (Dec.): 320–24.

Xiangshanxian zhi (Gazetteer of Xiangshan county). 1923. Li Shijin (comp.).

Xie Xingyao. 1950. *Taiping tianguo qianhou Guangxi de fan Qing yundong* (The anti-Qing movement in Guangxi before and after the Taiping Rebellion). Beijing: Sanlian shudian.

Xinan biancheng Mianning wuzhang (Five chapters on the southwestern border town of Mianning). 1937. Peng Gui'e (comp.).

Xingrenxian bu zhi (Amended gazetteer of Xingren county). 1943. Xingrenxian dang'an guan (comp.).

Xingrenxian zhi (Gazetteer of Xingren county). 1934. Ran Jing (comp.).

Xinpingxian zhi (Gazetteer of Xinping county). 1934. Wu Yongli (comp.).

(Xinsuan) Yunnan tongzhi (Revised comprehensive gazetteer of Yunnan). 1949. Long Yun (comp.).

Xinyifu zhi (Gazetteer of Xinyi prefecture). 1854. Zhang Ying (comp.).

(Xu) Mengzixian zhi (Revised gazetteer of Mengzi county). 1961 [1911]. Yi Ming (comp.).

Xu Wenbi. 1976 [Qing]. *Lizhi xuanjing* (A mirror of county administration). Taibei: Guangwen shuju.

(Xu) Yunnan tongzhigao (Revised comprehensive gazetteer of Yunnan). 1901. Wang Wenshao (comp.).

(Xuantong) Gaoyaoxian zhi ([Xuantong] gazetteer of Gaoyao county). 1938. Ma Chengtu (comp.).

Xundianzhou zhi (Gazetteer of Xundian department. 1828. Sun Shirong (comp.).

(*Xuxiu*) *Baiyanjing zhi* (Revised gazetteer of Baiyanjing). 1907 [1901]. Li Xuntuo (comp.).

(*Xuxiu*) *Jianshuixian zhigao* (Revised gazetteer of Jianshui county). 1920. Ding Guoliang (comp.).

(*Xuxiu*) *Menghua zhiliting zhi* (Revised gazetteer of Menghua autonomous subprefecture). 1790. Liu Kai (comp.).

(*Xuxiu*) *Songmingzhou zhi* (Revised gazetteer of Songming department. 1887. Hu Xuchang (comp.).

(*Xuxiu*) *Yongbei zhiliting zhi* (Revised gazetteer of Yongbei autonomous subprefecture). 1904. Ye Rutong (comp.).

Yanfengxian zhi (Gazetteer of Yanfeng county). 1924. Guo Xiexi (comp.).

Yang Shangchi. 1988. "30 niandai de quanguo haigang jianyi guanlichu yu Wu Liande boshi" (Dr. Wu Lien-teh and the nation's harbor quarantine stations in the 1930's). *Zhonghua yishi zazhi* (Journal of Chinese medical history) 18, no. 1: 29–32.

———. 1990. "Wo guo shouhui jianyi zhuquan de douzheng" (The struggle for regaining the right of quarantine). *Zhonghua yishi zazhi* (Journal of Chinese medical history) 20, no. 1: 25–27.

Yangjiangxian zhi (Gazetteer of Yangjiang county). 1925. Zhang Yicheng (comp.).

Yaoanxian zhi (Gazetteer of Yaoan county). 1948. Huo Shilian (comp.).

Yaozhou zhi (Gazetteer of Yaozhou department). 1885. Lu Songzheng (comp.).

Yiliangxian zhi (Gazetteer of Yiliang county). 1921. Wang Huairong (comp.).

Yongchangfu zhi (Gazetteer of Yongchang prefecture). 1826. Chen Tingyu (comp.).

Yongchangfu zhi (Gazetteer of Yongchang prefecture). 1885. Liu Yuke (comp.).

Yu Yongmin. 1989. "Qingmo Minguo shiqi Liaoning yiyao weisheng shilue." (A historical review of medical and health work in Liaoning province, 1881–1949). *Zhonghua yishi zazhi* (Journal of Chinese medical history) 19, no. 4: 193–99.

Yu Yue. 1935. *Quyuan biji* (Brush Sketches of Qu Garden). 2 vols. Shanghai: Dada tushu gongyingshe.

Yuan Shikai. 1971. *Yuan Shikai zuozhe zhuanji* (The memorials of Yuan Shikai). 8 vols. Taibei: Guoli gugong bowuyuan.

Yuan Wenkui. 1900 [1800]. *Guochao Diannan shilue* (Anthology of Qing poems from Yunnan). Wuhua shuyuan.

Yuanjiang zhigao (Gazetteer of Yuanjiang). 1922. Huang Yuanzhi (comp.).

Yulinzhou zhi (Gazetteer of Yulin department). 1894. Feng Decai (comp.).

Yunlongzhou zhi (Gazetteer of Yunlong department). 1892. Zhang Depei (comp.).

Yunnan tongzhi (Comprehensive gazetteer of Yunnan). 1894. Cen Yuying (comp.).

Yunnansheng lishi yanjiusuo (The Historical Research Institute of Yunnan Province). 1984. *"Qing shilu" you guan Yunnan shiliao huibian* (Historical materials concerning Yunnan in the *Qing Shilu* [Veritable records of the Qing]). 4 vols. Kunming: Renmin chubanshe.

Yunnanxian zhi (Gazetteer of Yunnan county). 1890. Xiang Lianjin (comp.).

(*Zengxiu*) *Renhuaiting zhi* (Revised gazetteer of Renhuai subprefecture). 1902. Zhang Zhengfeng (comp.).

Zhang Haipeng. 1983. *Zhongguo jindai shigao ditu ji.* (Atlas of modern Chinese history). Shanghai: Ditu chubanshe.

Zhang Renqun. 1967 [1897]. *Guangdong yudi quantu* (Comprehensive atlas of Guangdong province). Taibei: Chengwen chubanshe.

Zhang Yingchang. 1960 [1875]. *Qingshiduo* (Anthology of poems from the Qing period). 2 vols. Beijing: Zhonghua Shuju.

Zhang Yuanqi. 1911. *Dongsansheng yishi baogaoshu* (Report on the epidemic in the Three Eastern Provinces). Provincial Library of Taiwan. Photocopy.

Zhanyizhou zhi (Gazetteer of Zhanyi department). 1885. Chen Yan (comp.).

Zhao Yi. 1979. "Qiantan Ye Tianshi 'Wen re lun'" (A brief discussion of Ye Tianshi's *Wen re lun* [Treatise on Warm Factor disorders]). *Zhejiang zhongyiyao* (Chinese medicine in Zhejiang) 7: 240–42.

Zhao Yongling. 1982. "Jiashu shuyi" (Plague in commensal rats). *Yunnan yiyao* (Yunnan medicine) 5: 257–66.

Zhao Yongling and Yang Xiaodong. 1983. "Yunnan shuyi ziran yiyuandi fenbu de tantao" (An inquiry into the distribution of the natural plague foci in Yunnan). *Yunnan yiyao* (Yunnan medicine) 2: 108–9, 113.

Zhaotong zhigao (Gazetteer of Zhaotong). 1924. Fu Tingquan (comp.).

Zhejiangsheng zhongyi yanjiusuo (Zhejiang Chinese Medicine Research Institute). 1976. "*Wenyi lun*" *pingzhu* (Annotations on the "Discourse on heat epidemics"). Beijing: Renmin weisheng chubanshe.

Zheng Xiaoyan. 1936 [1901]. "Shuyi yuebian" (A brief treatise on plague). In Qiu Jisheng, ed., *Zhenben yishu ji cheng* (Collection of precious medical writings). Vol. 7. Shanghai: Shijie shuju.

Zhennanzhou zhi lue (Gazetteer of Zhennan department). 1892. Li Yulan (comp.).

Zhenxiongzhou zhi (Gazetteer of Zhenxiong department). 1887. Wu Guanghan (comp.).

Zhongyi yanjiuyuan (Chinese Academy of Traditional Chinese Medicine). Zhongguo yishi wenxian yanjiusuo (Division for research on historical documents on Chinese medicine). 1988. *Zhongyi renwu cidian* (Dictionary of notable figures in Chinese medicine). Shanghai: Shanghai cishu.

Ziegler, Philip. 1969. *The Black Death.* London: Collins.

Zongli Yamen Archives. Institute of Modern History, Academia Sinica, Taibei (Box on epidemic prevention and relief).

CHARACTER LISTS

Names, Terms, and Titles

Aiyu shantang　愛育善堂
awei　阿魏

ba gang　八綱
Bao Gong　包公
bianzheng lunzhi　辨證論治
bingyin　病因
Bo Lin　伯麟

caolongchuan　草龍船
Cen Chunxuan　岑春烜
Cen Yuying　岑育英
Chao Yuanfang　巢元方
Chenghuang shen　城隍神
Cixi　慈禧

Da Qing huidian　大清會典
Dantuxian zhi　丹徒縣志
dashi zhi　大事志
dayi　大疫
di qi　地氣
Dianshizhai huabao　點石齋畫報
Dongfang zazhi　東方雜誌
Donghua (Tung Wah)　東華
Du Wenxiu　杜文秀
Duanwu　端午

e'he　惡核

Fan Xingzhun　範行準
Fangyi zongju　防疫總局
fuji　扶乩

Gangyi　剛毅
Gongzhongdang　宮中檔
Gu Chun (Xihan)　顧純 (希翰)
Guandi (Guan Yu)　關帝 (關羽)
Guangji shantang　廣濟善堂
Gui Fang　桂芳
Gujin tushu ji cheng　古今圖書集成
guojia yixue　國家醫學

Han Guojun　韓國鈞
hezheng　核症
Hong Liangji (Beijiang)　洪亮吉
　(北江)
Hu Zhengxin　胡正心
Huang Daxian (Wong Tai Sin)
　黃大仙
Huang Liuhong (Huang Liu-hung)
　黃六鴻
Huang Zhongxian　黃仲賢
Huangdi neijing　黃帝內經
Huidian　會典
huiguan　會館

jiao　醮
Jiaoshe si　交涉司

jin　斤
Jingwu gongsuo　警務公所
Jiuhuang beilan　救荒備覽
Junji chu　軍機處
juren　舉人

Kang Da Yuanshuai　康大元帥
Kang Youwei　康有為

Lao Tong　勞潼
Le shantang (Lok-shin-tong)
　樂善堂
Li Hanzhang　李瀚章
li qi　戾氣
Li Shiyao　李侍堯
Li Xingrui　李興銳
Libu　禮部
ligui　癘鬼
lijin　釐金
Linshi fangyi hui　臨時防疫會
Litan　灉壇
Liu Binggua　劉秉括
liu jing　六經
liu qi　六氣
Liu Weichuan (Lau Wai Chuen)
　劉渭川
liu yin　六淫
Luo Fang　羅方
Luo Rulan (Zhiyuan)　羅汝蘭
　(芝園)

Ma Rulong　馬如龍
Mingde　明德
Mingshi　明史
Mingzheng si　民政司

Neige　內閣
Neijing　內經
Neizheng lei　內政類
Nongwu hui　農務會

Peng Ling　彭齡
ping'an dan　平安丹
pingmin weisheng　貧民衛生
puji tang　普濟堂

qi　氣
qi qing　七情
Qian jin fang　千金方
qihou　氣候
Qing Bao　慶保
Qing jiao　清醮
Qingshi liezhuan　清史列傳
Qu Yuan　屈原

Renji shantang　仁濟善堂

sanjiao　三焦
shanghan　傷寒
Shanghan lun　傷寒論
Shangwu zonghui　商務總會
shantang　善堂
Shengjing shibao　盛京時報
Shi Daonan　師道南
Shi Fan　師範
shiyao ju　施藥局
shuyi　鼠疫
Shuyi fei yi—liu jing tiaobian
　鼠疫非疫—六經條辨
Shuyi huibian　鼠疫彙編
Shuyi yuebian　鼠疫約編
Siji ru chun　四季如春
Simiao shantang　司廟善堂 [?]
songwen　送瘟
sou yi　搜疫

Taihe yiju　太和醫局
Taiping tianguo　太平天國
Taiyiyuan　太醫院
Tan Congchan　譚聰產
Tang Sunhua　唐孫華
tenghuang　膽黃
tian qi　天氣
Tian xing yi guo　天行已過
Tian yu ji　天禹集
Tong shantang　同善堂

wai yin　外因
Wang jiao　王醮
wei qi ying xue　衛氣營血
Weisheng fangyi zhan　衛生防疫站

Weisheng ke   衛生科
Weisheng si   衛生司
Wen Chang   文昌
Wen Yuanshuai   溫元帥
wenbing   瘟病 (溫病)
Wenbu   瘟部
wenchuan   瘟船
Wenjiao lei   文教類
wenshen   瘟神
wenshen jiao   瘟神醮
wenyi   瘟疫
Wenyi lun   瘟疫論
Wu Dacheng   吳大澂
Wu Tang (Jutong)   吳塘 (鞠通)
Wu Youxing (Youke)   吳有性
    (又可)
Wu Zongxuan (Xuecun)   吳宗宣
    (學存)
Wuwen shizhe   五瘟使者
wuxing   五行
Wuzazu   五雜俎

xiangyi   祥異
xie qi   邪氣
Xie Zhaozhi   謝肇制
Xiliang   錫良
Xin Zhu   新柱
xinzheng   新政
Xu Naiji   許乃濟
Xu Shichang   徐世昌
Xu Yingkui   許應騤
xuezheng   學正

yangzibing   瘍子病
yaofang   藥方
Ye Gui (Tianshi)   葉桂 (天士)
yi   疫
yi an   醫案

yi qi liuxing   疫氣流行
yigui   疫鬼
yinyang   陰陽
yiyao weisheng   醫藥衛生
Yuan Shikai   袁世凱
Yuan Tang   袁棠
Yuan Wenkui   袁文揆
Yuan Yixiang   袁一相

zaixiang   災祥
zangfu   臟腑
Zhang Ji (Zhongjing)   張機 (仲景)
Zhang Shicheng   張師誠
Zhang Yingchang   張應昌
Zhang Yuanqi   張元奇
zhangqi   瘴氣
Zhao Erxun   趙爾巽
zhen qi   眞氣
zheng qi   正氣
Zheng Xiaoyan   鄭肖岩
zheng1   症
zheng2   證
zhenji   賑濟
Zhi shuyi fa   治鼠疫法
Zhongguo shuyi liuxingshi
    中國鼠疫流行史
Zhongyi renwu cidian
    中醫人物詞典
Zhou Shanpei   周善培
Zhou Sicheng   周思程
zhu yi   逐疫
Zhu yigui   逐疫鬼
Zhubing yuanhou zonglun
    諸病源侯總論
zhuo qi   濁氣
Zhupi zouzhe   朱批奏摺
Zizhi hui   自治會
Zuo zhuan   左傳

Place Names

This character list includes only names in Mandarin Chinese and only those place names mentioned in the text, tables, or maps. (Thus Vietnamese names such as Haiphong and Hanoi are not included, nor are the Cantonese or English names of districts of Hong Kong.) Place names that only occur in gazetteer titles are not necessarily included. Rivers and provinces are not included. Most administrative units are identified by the name in use during the late Qing period. Current designations are listed in parentheses for those places whose names have been changed since the nineteenth century. An asterisk indicates those few cases where only new (post-1949) names are used. Abbreviations in brackets refer to the following provinces:

[FJ]	Fujian	[JS]	Jiangsu
[FT]	Fengtian (Liaoning)	[JL]	Jilin
[GD]	Guangdong	[SC]	Sichuan
[GX]	Guangxi	[TW]	Taiwan
[GZ]	Guizhou	[YN]	Yunnan
[HL]	Heilongjiang	[ZJ]	Zhejiang
[HB]	Hubei	[ZL]	Zhili (Hebei)
[HN]	Hunan		

Adunzi [YN]　阿墩子
Agou subprefecture [TW]　阿狗廳
Ami department (Kaiyuan) [YN]　阿迷州 (開遠)
Anning department [YN]　安寧州
Anping county [GZ]　安平縣
Anpu [GD]　安浦
Anren county [HN]　安仁縣

Anshun county [GZ]　安順縣
Anxi county [FJ]　安溪縣
Aomen (Macao)　奧門

Baishan township [GX]　白山司
Baiyanjing county (Yanfeng) [YN]　白鹽井縣 (鹽豐)
Baoshan county [YN]　保山縣

Baoshan prefecture [YN]　保山府
Beihai (Pakhoi) [GD]　北海
Beijing [ZL]　北京
Beiliu county [GX]　北流縣
Binchuan department [YN]
　賓川州
Binzhou department (Binyang)
　[GX]　賓州(賓陽)
Bobai county [GX]　博白縣
Bose subprefecture [GX]　百色廳

Changchun [JL]　長春
Changle county [FJ]　長樂縣
Changning* county [YN]　昌寧縣
Changsha [HN]　長沙
Changtai county [FJ]　長泰縣
Changzhou prefecture [JS]
　長州府
Chaoyang county [GD]　潮陽縣
Chaozhou prefecture [GD]
　潮州府
Chengdu [SC]　成都
Chenggong county [YN]　呈貢縣
Chenghai county [GD]　澂海縣
Chengmai county [GD]　澄邁縣
Chongan county [FJ]　崇安縣
Chongbaosha Island [JS]
　崇寶沙島
Chongqing [SC]　重慶
Chongshan county [GX]　崇善縣
Chuxiong county [YN]　楚雄縣
Chuxiong prefecture [YN]　楚雄府
Chuzhou prefecture [ZJ]　處州府
Conghua county [GD]　從化縣

Dali county [YN]　大理縣
Dali prefecture [YN]　大理府
Danxian [GD]　儋縣
Dapu county [GD]　大埔縣
Datian county [FJ]　大田縣
Dehong autonomous department
　[YN]　德宏直隸州
Dengchuan department [YN]
　燈川州
Dianbai county [GD]　電白縣

Dianchi Lake [YN]　滇池
Diannan　滇南
Dingan county [GD]　定安縣
Dongchuan prefecture [YN]
　東川府
Dongguan county [GD]　東莞縣
Dongmen county [JS]　東門縣
Dongshan Island [FJ]　東山島
Douliu subprefecture [TW]
　斗六廳

Er'hai Lake [YN]　洱海

Fanshucai subprefecture [TW]
　藩薯蔡廳
Fengshan subprefecture [TW]
　鳳山廳
Fengshun county [GD]　豐順縣
Fengtian prefecture [FT]　奉天府
Foshan county [GD]　佛山縣
Fuan prefecture [FJ]　福安府
Fumin county [YN]　富民縣
Fuqing county [FJ]　福清縣
Fuzhou (Foochow) [FJ]　福州

Gaoyao county (Zhaoqing) [GD]
　高要縣(肇慶)
Gaozhou prefecture [GD]　高州府
Gejiu [YN]　個舊
Guangnan county (Baoning) [YN]
　廣南縣(寶寧)
Guangnan prefecture [YN]
　廣南府
Guangning county [GD]　廣寧縣
Guangtong county (Mouding) [YN]
　廣通縣(牟定)
Guangze county [FJ]　光澤縣
Guangzhou (Canton) [GD]　廣州
Guiping county [GX]　桂平縣
Guixian county [GX]　貴縣
Guiyang prefecture [GZ]　貴陽府
Gutian county [FJ]　古田縣

Haicheng county (Longhai) [FJ]
　海澄縣(龍海)

Luzhou [SC]　瀘州

Maguan* county [YN]　馬關縣
Malipo* [YN]　麻栗坡
Malong department [YN]　馬龍州
Manhao [YN]　蠻耗
Manzhouli [HL]　滿州里
Meizhou prefecture [GD]　梅州府
Menghua autonomous subprefecture [YN]　蒙化直隸廳
Mengzi county [YN]　蒙自縣
Mianning subprefecture (Lancang) [YN]　緬寧廳
Miaoli subprefecture [TW]　苗栗廳
Midu county [YN]　彌渡縣
Mile county [YN]　彌勒縣
Minbei　閩北
Minnan　閩南
Minqing county [FJ]　閩清縣
Minxian county [FJ]　閩縣

Nan'an county [FJ and YN]　南安縣
Nanhai county [GD]　南海縣
Nanjing county [FJ]　南靖縣
Nanning county (Qujing) [YN]　南寧縣 (曲靖)
Nanning prefecture [GX]　南寧府
Nanping county [FJ]　南平縣
Nantou subprefecture [TW]　南投廳
Ningbo (Ningpo) [ZJ]　寧波
Ningde county [FJ]　寧德縣
Ning'er county (Pu'er) [YN]　寧洱縣 (普洱)
Ningzhou department (Huaning) [YN]　寧州 (華寧)

Panyu county [GD]　番愚縣
Penghu subprefecture [TW]　澎湖廳
Pinghe county [FJ]　平和縣
Pingle prefecture [GX]　平樂府
Pingnan county [GX]　平南縣
Pingnan county [FJ]　屏南縣

Pingtan county [FJ]　平潭縣
Pingxiang minority department [GX]　憑祥土州
Pingyuan county [GD]　平遠縣
Pucheng county [FJ]　浦城縣
Pu'er prefecture [YN]　普洱府
Puning county [GD]　普寧縣
Pupiao [YN]　蒲漂
Putian county [FJ]　莆田縣

Qianjiang county [GX]　遷江縣
Qingyuan county [GD]　慶遠縣
Qingyuan prefecture [GX]　慶遠府
Qinzhou [GD]　欽州
Qiongshan county [GD]　瓊山縣
Qiubei county [YN]　邱北縣
Quanzhou [FJ]　泉州
Qujing prefecture [YN]　曲靖府

Raoping county [GD]　饒平縣
Rongxian [GX]　容縣
Ruili* county [YN]　瑞麗縣

Shanglin county [GX]　上林縣
Shantou (Swatow) [GD]　汕頭
Shaowu county [FJ]　邵武縣
Shaowu prefecture [FJ]　邵武府
Shaoxing prefecture [ZJ]　紹興府
Shaozhou prefecture [GD]　韶州府
Shaxian county [FJ]　沙縣
Shenkeng subprefecture [TW]　深坑廳
Shenyang (Mukden) [FT]　沈陽
Shicheng county (Lianjiang) [GD]　石城縣 (廉江)
Shidian county (Changning) [YN]　施甸縣 (昌寧)
Shiping county [YN]　石屏縣
Shunchang county [FJ]　順昌縣
Shunde county [GD]　順得縣
Shunning prefecture (Fengqing) [YN]　順寧府 (風慶)
Simao subprefecture [YN]　思矛廳
Songming department [YN]　嵩明州

Songxi county [FJ]　松溪縣
Suixi county [GD]　遂溪縣

Taibei subprefecture [TW]　台北廳
Taidong subprefecture [TW]
　台東廳
Tainan subprefecture [TW]
　台南廳
Taining county [FJ]　泰寧縣
Taiping prefecture [GX]　太平府
Taipingshan　太平山
Taishan county [GD]　台山縣
Taizhong subprefecture [TW]
　台中廳
Taizhou prefecture [ZJ]　台州府
Talang subprefecture (Mojiang)
　[YN]　他郎廳(墨江)
Taoyuan subprefecture [TW]
　桃園廳
Tengchong* county [YN]　騰沖縣
Tengxian county [GX]　藤縣
Tengyue subprefecture (Tengchong)
　[YN]　騰越廳 (騰沖)
Tianjin (Tientsin) [ZL]　天津
Tianyang department [GX]
　田陽州
Tingzhou prefecture [FJ]　汀州府
Tongan county [FJ]　同安縣
Tonghai county [YN]　通海縣
Tongzhou department [ZL]　通州

Weining department [GZ]　威寧州
Weishan* county [YN]　巍山縣
Wenshan county (Kaihua) [YN]
　文山縣 (開化)
Wenzhou [ZJ]　溫州
Wuchuan county [GD]　吳川縣
Wuhua* county [GD]　五化縣
Wusong [JS]　吳松
Wuyi Mountains　武夷山
Wuyuan county (Wuming) [GX]
　武緣縣 (武鳴)
Wuzhou [GX]　梧州

Xiaguan county [YN]　下關縣

Xiamen (Amoy) [FJ]　廈門
Xianggang (Hong Kong)　香港
Xiangshan county (Zhongshan)
　[GD]　香山縣 (中山)
Xiangyun* county [YN]　祥雲縣
Xianyou county [FJ]　仙游縣
Xiapu county [FJ]　霞浦縣
Xi'e county (Eshan) [YN]　嵋峨縣
　(峨山)
Xigang [TW]　西港
Xilin county [GX]　西林縣
Xincheng [GD]　新城
Xingning county [GD]　興寧縣
Xingyi prefecture [GZ]　興義府
Xinhui county [GD]　新會縣
Xinping county [YN]　新平縣
Xinxing county [GD]　新興縣
Xinxing department (Yuxi) [YN]
　新興州(玉溪)
Xinyi county [GD]　信宜縣
Xinzhu subprefecture [TW]
　新竹廳
Xishuangbanna* [YN]　西雙版納
Xiyingpan (Saiyingpun)　西營盤
Xuanwei department [YN]
　宣威州
Xundian department [YN]　尋甸州
Xunzhou prefecture [GX]　潯州府
Xuwen county [GD]　徐聞縣
Xuyong prefecture [SC]　敘永府
Xuzhou department (Yibin) [SC]
　敘州 (宜賓)

Yangjiang autonomous subprefec-
　ture [GD]　陽江直隸廳
Yanglin county [YN]　楊林縣
Yangtangli [YN]　羊塘里
Yanping prefecture [FJ]　延平府
Yangzhou [JS]　楊州
Yanshuigang subprefecture [TW]
　鹽水港廳
Yaozhou department (Yaoan) [YN]
　姚州(姚安)
Yilan subprefecture [TW]　宜蘭廳
Yiliang county [YN]　彝良縣

Yingjiang county [YN]　盈江縣
Yingkou (Newchang) [FT]　營口
Yizheng [JS]　依征
Yongan county [FJ]　永安縣
Yongan county (Zijin) [GD]　永安縣(紫金)
Yongbei autonomous subprefecture [YN]　永北直隸廳
Yongchang prefecture (Baoshan) [YN]　永昌府 (保山)
Yongchun county [FJ]　永春縣
Yongding county [FJ]　永定縣
Yongfu county (Yongtai) [FJ]　永福縣 (永泰)
Yongjia county (Wenzhou) [ZJ]　永嘉縣 (溫州)
Yongping county [YN]　永平縣
Youxi county [FJ]　尤溪縣
Yuanjiang autonomous department [YN]　元江直隸州
Yulin county [GX]　玉林縣
Yungui　雲貴
Yunlong department [YN]　雲龍州
Yunnan county (Xiangyun) [YN]　雲南縣 (祥雲)
Yunnan prefecture (Kunming) [YN]　雲南府 (昆明)
Yunxiao subprefecture [FJ]　雲霄廳

Zengcheng county [GD]　增城縣
Zhanghua subprefecture [TW]　彰化廳
Zhangping county [FJ]　漳平縣
Zhangpu county [FJ]　漳浦縣
Zhangquan [FJ]　漳泉
Zhangzhou [FJ]　漳州
Zhanjiang [GD]　湛江
Zhanyi department [YN]　沾益州
Zhaoan county [FJ]　詔安縣
Zhaoqing prefecture [GD]　肇慶府
Zhaotong county (En'an)　昭通縣 (恩安)
Zhaotong prefecture [YN]　昭通府
Zhaozhou county [YN]　趙州縣
Zhenghe county [FJ]　政和縣
Zhennan department (Nanhua) [YN]　鎮南州 (南華)
Zhenping county (Jiaoling) [GD]　鎮平縣 (蕉嶺)
Zhenxiong department [YN]　鎮雄州
Zhenzhou department (Yuanling) [HN]　振州 (元陵)
Zhongdian subprefecture [YN]　中甸廳
Zhoudun county (Zhouning) [FJ]　周墩縣 (周寧)

INDEX

Index

In this index an "f" after a number indicates a separate reference on the next page, and an "ff" indicates separate references on the next two pages. A continuous discussion over two or more pages is indicated by a span of page numbers, e.g., "57–58." *Passim* is used for a cluster of references in close but not continuous sequence.

250   Index

Longan county (Guangxi), 1864 epidemic
in, 62
Longxi county (Fujian), plague in, 87
Longzhou (Guangxi), 54, 60, 62, 196n5,
208n9
Lowson, Dr. James, 141
Luchuan county (Guangdong), 1888
epidemic in, 70
Lufeng county (Yunnan), 41
Luo Fang, 135
Luo Rulan (Luo Zhiyuan), 107ff, 201n10
Luoping department (Yunnan), 53
Luoyuan county (Fujian), plague in, 90
Luzhou (Sichuan), 27

Ma Rulong, 39
Macao, 1895 epidemic in, 203n20
McNeill, William, 10, 50
Macroregions, in 19th-century China, 11–
13. *See also individual macroregions by
name*
Madah, 28
Maguan (Yunnan), 1865–66 epidemic in,
60
Malaria, 17f, 55, 119, 123, 180, 182, 186–87,
192n3
Malipo (Yunnan), 1866 epidemic in, 60
Manchuria, 6, 14, 151, 156; pneumonic
plague epidemic of 1910–11 in, 6, 151,
155–63, 167–68, 171, 203n22, 208n10,
209n19
Manchurian Plain, 6
Manchurian railway, 156, 167
Manchus, 28, 162
Mandalay, 28
Manhao (Yunnan), 53, 197n9
Mann, Susan, 193n9
Manzhouli, 1910 epidemic in, 156
Marine Hospital Service, *see* United States
Public Health Service
Marmota sibirica (Siberian marmot or
tarbagan), 156. *See also* Plague, vectors
of
Marseilles, 1720–22 epidemic in, 77f
Marshall Wen, *see* Wen Yuanshuai
Measles, 76
Medical geography, 11, 73–76
Medical police, 154, 156ff. See also Police,
new-style; Public health, police-
directed model of

Mediterranean: 6th- and 14th-century
epidemics in, 1; 1720–22 epidemic in,
77
Menghua autonomous subprefecture
(Yunnan): 1776 epidemic in, 30; 1846–
47 epidemic in, 33, 39; 1854–62 epidemics in, 42
Mengzi county (Yunnan), 21, 28, 48, 53ff,
60, 117, 120f; 1812 epidemic in, 32;
1873–93 epidemics in, 45f
Meningeal plague, 4. *See also* Plague,
forms of
Mianning subprefecture (Yunnan), 1854–
62 epidemics in, 42
Miasmas, 100, 111, 140. See also *Zhangqi*
Miasmatic theory of infectious disease,
105, 108f, 130, 139f
Microbiological revolution (1880s–1890s),
138, 169. *See also* Germ theory of disease
Microbiology, 168
Middle East, 9, 100f, 128f, 205n38; 6th-
and 14th-century epidemics in, 1
Min River, 80f, 83, 90, 92, 198n1
Minbei, 83
Ming dynasty, transport routes in Yunnan
during, 27, 194n14
Ming-Qing transition, 9f, 25
Mingde, 124
Mingshi (Ming history), 10
Ministry of Epidemics (Wenbu), 110, 113,
119f
Minnan, 83
Minxian (Fujian), 107
Mongolia, 156, 167
Mongols, road construction in Yunnan by,
194n14
Morbidity: of disease, 75f, 97f; of plague,
175–76
Mortality, *see* Plague, mortality due to.
See also Plague, demographic impact of
Mus musculus (common house mouse), 81,
199n6. *See also* Plague, vectors of
Muslim Rebellion (1856–73), 37–50 *passim*,
59f, 119, 166f, 194n14, 197n9, 204n30
Muslims, 39, 41, 50, 59, 129f, 160

Nanhai county (Guangdong), 1894 epidemic in, 206n1
Nanning prefecture (Guangxi), 28, 51–58
passim, 62, 65, 195n17, 196n4

Naples, 77f
Naquin, Susan, 194n12
New Mexico, plague in, 193n7
New Policy (*xinzheng*) Reforms, 3, 150f,
163f, 166
New York Times, 193n7
Niles, Mary, 135
Ningbo (Ningpo), 152
Ningde county (Fujian), plague in, 90
Ning'er county (Yunnan), 1860 and 1862
epidemics in, 43, 45
Norris, John, 10, 166
North China Herald, 134, 147
North Manchurian Plague Prevention
Service, 164, 192n7.
Nu (Salween) River, 21, 50
Number One Historical Archives, Beijing,
122

Old age as cause of death, 186f
Opium trade: domestic, 3, 50–59 *passim*,
71, 167, 196n6, 198n15; foreign, 51, 55f,
196n5; Yunnan, 35, 51ff, 59f, 70, 195n17,
196n5, 196–97n8. *See also* Yunnan-
Lingnan, opium trade
Opium War, 131
Orientalism, 169
Orthopathic *qi* (*zhengqi*) 102f, 105
Ou River, 80, 198n1

Pandemics of plague, 1
Panyu county (Guangdong), 1894 epi-
demic in, 206n1
Pasteurella pestis, see *Yersinia pestis*
Pearl River Delta, 2, 49, 53, 57, 65, 70, 133,
196n4
People's Republic of China, 5, 11, 192n4;
Ministry of Health, 11
Persia, 205n34
Pestilential *qi* (*li qi*), 104, 106ff, 120
Pingle prefecture (Guangxi), 57
Pingtan Island (Fujian), 90
Pingxiang (Guangxi), 54, 197n10
Pirates, 56, 197n11
Plague: third (modern) pandemic, 1–3,
49f, 70, 80, 130, 165–69 *passim*, 195n22;
epidemiological research on, 2, 11,
14–15, 20–22, 45, 50, 60, 64, 108, 140–
41, 169; demographic impact of, 2f,
10, 75–77, 86, 96–99, 175; urban vs.

rural nature of, 3, 72, 76–80, 97; and
long-distance trade, 3–7 *passim*, 14, 25,
29–35, 47–51, 60, 65–71, 76–79, 96, 156,
165–68; diffusion of, 3, 35, 72, 76–98
passim; case-fatality rates of, 4, 22, 143,
147f, 170, 206n10, 207n12; epidemiology of, 4–5, 11, 20, 169, 191n2; forms
of, 4, 8, 10, 22, 24, 83, 151, 156; symptoms of, 4, 8ff, 14, 24, 40, 43, 128–29;
natural reservoirs of, 4–7, 11, 20–22, 24,
29, 47, 64–66 *passim*, 71, 156, 195n18;
treatment of, 4, 147; vectors (hosts) of,
4–7, 21f, 76f, 81–83, 156, 167, 193n7,
199n6; commensal foci of, 5ff, 21, 81;
ecology of 5–7, 11, 14, 20–22, 29, 47, 64–
65, 70–71, 81–83, 156; as metaphor, 7–8,
128; Chinese terminology for, 8, 14, 18–
19, 101, 128; in pre-Qing China, 9–11;
mortality due to, 24, 31ff, 40–46 *passim*,
62, 77, 86, 90, 142f, 156, 175–78, 193n10;
etiology, European beliefs about, 100,
108, 140–44, 169; etiology, Chinese
medical beliefs about, 100, 105–7, 129f;
communal responses to, 100–101, 115–
21, 128–30, 134, 165, 205n38; popular
Chinese beliefs about, 110–15; official Qing responses to, 122–28, 130,
133–34, 157–64 *passim*, 170–71, 203–6;
20th-century control measures, 169, 175
Plague demons (ghosts), see *Yigui*
Plague gods, see *Wenshen*
Plague of Justinian, 1
Plagues and Peoples, 50
Planchette (*fuji*), 112ff, 119f
Pneumonia, 186f
Pneumonic plague, *see* Plague, forms of.
See also under India; Manchuria
Poland, 14th-century epidemic in, 1
Police: and public health, 151, 154–55,
163f, 166, 171; in Shenyang during
1910–11 epidemic, 151, 157–59; new-
style, 151–57 *passim*, 163, 171, 208n7;
Daotai system (*Jingwu gongsuo*), 155,
208n9
Pollitzer, R., 50, 79f, 88
Pregnancy and childbirth, mortality in,
186f
Proportionate mortality ratio (PMR), 180,
187
Prussian mercantilism, 154

Library of Congress Cataloging-in-Publication Data

Benedict, Carol (Carol Ann)
 Bubonic plague in nineteenth-century China / Carol Benedict.
  p.   cm.
 Includes bibliographical references and index.
 ISBN 0-8047-2661-2 (cloth)
  1. Plague—China—History—19th century.   I. Title.
RC179.C6B46   1996
614.5'732'0095109034—dc20   96-5157
                                                              CIP

Original printing 1996
Last figure below indicates year of this printing:

05   04   03   02   01   00   99   98   97   96

⊛   This book is printed on acid-free, recycled paper.